REAL

FOOD

Reset

30 days to lose weight, be free from cravings & feeling great!

Get in touch with your primal instincts, detox your body, and cleanse yourself of cravings, with real food even paleo man would enjoy!

Galina Ivanova Denzel, NSCA-CPT, Restorative Exercise Specialist, Somatic Experience Therapist

Roland Denzel, IKFF-CKT, Precision Nutrition

Fit Ink Publications

Praise for The REAL FOOD Reset

"Are you ready to jumpstart your way to vibrant energy and better health? Roland and Galina Denzel have written a concise but powerful guide to improving your life with nature's most powerful medicine – real food.

All too often, our Standard American Diet leaves us overfed but undernourished. *The Real Food Reset* will teach you how to make real, unprocessed food the cornerstone of your comprehensive plan to improve the quality of your life..."

– Wendy Welch, MD, WendyWellness.com

"*The Real Food Reset* is a very simple to follow plan that is presented in a straight-forward and pleasant manner. It doesn't make itself out to be more than it is or bog itself down with meaningless information or pseudo-science.

The book is quick to the point and gives the reader everything they need to formulate their own dietary plan and even provides a tracking system to quantify the positive effects that are occurring that might otherwise be overlooked.

After the 30 days the reader will have the education and practice to carry the plan forward forever."

– Anthony Sayers, NASM-CPT, PES

Updates

For free updates on this book and our other projects, sign up at EatMoveLive52.com/Contact.

You'll get access to free book and recipe resources, plus be the first to know about our upcoming projects!

Table of Contents

Introduction 1

Detoxes, cleanses, and other magic 3

It's a miracle! 3

Clean as you go 3

Wouldn't it be fantastic 5

The downside to being human 6

Species-specific 9

Do we love our animals more than we love ourselves? 10

Gorillas in the midst 11

'I'm not an animal, I'm a human being.' 12

YOU on a [human] DIET 13

Fat, sick, and ready to believe it's inevitable 21

The new normal 23

Like father like son 23

Overriding your instincts 24

The Real Food Reset 26

It really works! 27

Get your mind on board 28

The empty promise 29

The big button reset 31

It's all about the [real] food 32

Good Guys (eat these) 33

Bad Guys (don't eat these) 35

Let's do this! 40

Focus on these foods.. *40*

Completely avoid these foods *49*

Minimize these foods *50*

Avoid these foods if you have allergies............................. *51*

Planning and preparing... **55**

Pantry and fridge clean up.. *55*

To the store!.. *56*

Plan your menu *57*

How to build a meal... *59*

All things NOT food.. **71**

Sleep.. *71*

Exercise *72*

Supplements *73*

How to track your weight progress.................................... *74*

How to track your 'health' progress *80*

30 Days of Real Food Symptom Tracker *81*

What if nothing is happening?.. *82*

Day 31 and beyond **84**

What happens if I stop dieting?... *84*

Can I reintroduce certain foods?... *85*

Come on, live a little! *91*

The 90% rule *93*

Maintenance (or, will this diet ever be done?) *98*

Have a plan *99*

Join the community **101**

Stay connected.. *101*

Acknowledgments **104**

Attributions *104*

Disclaimer

You must get your doctor's approval before beginning this diet and exercise program.

This book/ebook provides information that you read and use at your own risk. We do not take responsibility for any misfortune that may happen, either directly or indirectly, from reading and applying the information contained and/or referenced in this book/ebook. The programs and information expressed within this book/ebook are NOT medical advice, but rather represent the authors' opinions, and are solely for informational and educational purposes.

Please do not use the information in this book without first discussing your fitness, training, and nutrition plans with a qualified doctor or health practitioner. The authors are not responsible for any injury or health condition that may occur through following the programs and opinions expressed within this book. The dietary information is presented for informational purposes only and may not be appropriate for all individuals.

Remember; consult with your physician before starting any exercise program or altering your diet.

Introduction

We launched our *30 Days of Real Food* program on our website in January, and testimonials started coming in within a week – pain gone, energy returning, skin clearing, digestion improving.

People in our community online and in our small city in Southern California were onto something – by following a real food diet, one can undo months and years of poor dietary habits.

"I couldn't believe that in only 30 days I lost 15lbs, my hands felt free from arthritis, and I had energy to walk everywhere! It was so easy! Why didn't I do it earlier?" – Bryan, 35 years old

"I've had acne my whole life. In the back of my mind I always knew it might be food and I kind of suspected dairy. Since I cut it out, my skin is so much clearer. I also have energy the whole day and don't get sleepy at work at 4 p.m. This program has changed my life!" – Carolyne, 27 years old

"I dropped 5lbs the first week on the program. I didn't think it would be that easy. I am still losing weight, I started exercising again and I can play with my grandkids. My daughter is getting married in a week and I can't believe how in shape I am for her wedding!" – Johanna, 53 years old

"The 30 Days of Real Food has gone beyond our wildest expectations. I am a carb lover, everything from bread to French fries I love. With that, Sean and I didn't know how well we would do. We weren't perfect every day, but we tried our best. Our energy levels are through the roof, no more crashing in the afternoon, I have lost 12 pounds, our sleep has improved, we are able to be more active and have noticed we don't have to eat as much during the day. We plan to continue this for the most part after the 30 day challenge!" – Rosie and Sean, 30 years old

These are just some of the testimonials that our friends and readers have shared. When we started the '*30 Days of Real Food*,' it was a way to organize the advice that we give all our readers; eat food that is minimally processed, stay on track by having a clear goal, pay attention to rest and restoration, and move more.

Unlike a diet, a detox or a flush, after 30 days on Real Food, you will have developed healthy eating habits that can become a platform of perfect health for the rest of your life.

In your hands you are holding the book that will teach you everything you need to know about starting your own '30 Days,' how to keep your results, and continue to improve going forward.

Detoxes, cleanses, and other magic

It's a miracle!

Go on the Internet and do a simple search or, God forbid, get on the wrong spammer's email list, and you will be bombarded with thousands of 21 day detoxes, 7 day cleanses and magical, miracle diet plans.

They start with the infamous 'colon cleanse,' cruise through 'the liver protocol,' tempt you with the 'burns twice' feeling of cayenne pepper and lemonade tea, then onto diets of protein shakes or smoothies! They all promise to make you slimmer, give you more energy and prove to you that you can do it, if only you could stick to it, knuckle down, and possibly buy an industrial strength juicer or blender (only $599, plus shipping and handling)!

Clean as you go

"Wow. You know, it says here that by the time the average American is fifty, he's got five pounds of undigested red meat in his bowels." – Judge Reinhold, as Detective Rosewood in the classic 80s movie Beverly Hills Cop

We are a complicated species, and we've been around for a long time. The Earth is filled with complicated species other than ours, too. You don't see them detoxing, do you? They are not addicted to the high colonic.

Animals in the wild live long and healthy lives, accidents and predators aside, and so can we. ...all without worrying about 'cleansing our colons' and coffee enemas.

My friend Lou Schuler, writer and editor at Men's Health Magazine and author of some of our favorite fitness books, once researched what was behind (pun definitely intended) the idea of the colon cleanse, and its popularity. Turns out it all started with that one throwaway moment from the '80s classic movie Beverly Hills Cop.

"It's an entire industry built from a single line in Beverly Hills Cop. Bottom line, if it involves a body penetrating rubber hose in a non-medical setting, it's not a good idea." writes Lou in The New Rules of Lifting Supercharged.

We couldn't agree more.

Most people who have eaten corn, then looked at their next #2 before flushing, should realize that things simply don't stay in the body for very long. On average, what goes in, comes out, within about twenty four hours.

Cleansing and detoxing do occur, however, but it's happening 24/7, whether you eat or not. Chemicals go in via food, water, and air, and come out via feces, urine, sweat, and breath. Your body cleanses itself better than you ever could, provided you feed it the right stuff and don't overload it with too much to handle. In fact, since your body and your bodily functions (metabolism) run faster or slower depending on your level of food intake and activity, I'd have to say that eating a clean diet is critical to the very best detox or cleanse, and limiting yourself to a stripped down diet, devoid of nutrition (such as cabbage soup or detox tea) is the last thing you should do.

Wouldn't it be fantastic

...if you could eat a diet that ensures you would never again feel like you *needed* a detox?

It is possible that you feel you need a detox now, but step one isn't a detox; step one is taking a look at your plate.

The downside to being human

Is there really a downside to being human? Sure, we have to go to work, pay our taxes, and take out the garbage, but that's a small price to pay for all the fun and interesting things we get to do, like invent stuff, fall in love, race cars, vacation around the world, and argue on the Internet. We humans are in control of our lives to a large degree. We are conscious, and we make our own decisions! That's really awesome.

Yes, we've grown beyond reacting to our instincts, and now get to use our rational minds to control our destiny in ways that our animal friends can't. We can grow our own food, invent things to eat that our ancestors never dreamed of, and concoct medicines that try to fix all of our ailments. All good stuff, right?

Unfortunately, free will and inventiveness do not always lead to good things... Today's 'mom jeans' and the popular hairstyles from the '80s clearly show that we don't always make the best decisions. It's also pretty clear that it can take a while to realize our mistakes, and it's not just fashion where we blow it; one of the most glaring areas of opportunity is in fitness and nutrition.

We are in the midst of an obesity epidemic that is 100% our own making – even if it's not on purpose – and we're just starting to realize that our attempts to make life easier and tastier might be to blame.

Machines, computers, and modern day jobs leave us less active. Modern foods have been engineered to be tasty, cheap, and plentiful, and provide a lot more calories than most of us need to be eating today, considering our mostly sedentary lives.

As a result, we get fat, weak, and sick, and end up less healthy than our ancestors.

According to the CDC's National Center for Health Statistics we are living an average of 30 years longer since the 1900s, with 1.7% of us reaching ago 100 today compared to a mere .03% back in the 1900s (*CDC, MMWR, Vol 48/No 12, CDC 1999*).

We don't have to compare today to 110 years ago, either; our lifespans continue to increase year over year (*Arias E. United States life tables, 2008. National Vital Statistics Reports; vol 61 no 3. Hyattsville, MD: NCHS 2012.*), but how healthy are those last years?

There are arguments to be made that living longer gives us the chance to experience diseases and conditions that we would not have contracted in previous, shorter lived generations, but there are also those who believe that many of the 'diseases of age' are preventable, to some degree or another.

Still, healthy or sick, we are living longer than ever before, thanks to a medical community that struggles to fight off these plagues that we bring on ourselves rather than stop them before they start.

So what happened? Are we no longer listening to (or even hearing) our instincts? Do our instincts conspire against us?

No, we hear *and* we listen, but the same instincts that have helped us survive through famine, plague, and drought are the same ones that now work against our health and waistlines.

Our bodies are designed to prepare for the worst, and in anticipation of the worst (like starvation), they take every opportunity to store fat for an emergency.

Fortunately, in our modern world, it's rare to be subjected to famine. Unfortunately, our bodies don't know that, so they instinctively prepare for the famine that never comes.

So, why weren't our ancestors as fat as we are today? Easy calories, like cakes, breads, fast food, candies, packaged foods, and ice cream weren't nearly as easy to come by as they are today. In fact, long ago, only the wealthy were overweight, but we've made empty calories so inexpensive that anyone can be fat, today. Go equality!

Our bodies know easy calories, and condition our minds (via our instincts) to recognize them. When we see, smell, and taste them, we instinctively eat as much of them as we can, merely to store the energy (as fat) for later, rich or poor, famine or no famine.

Because our instincts lead us to tasty foods (because they know that's what stores fat and keeps us alive), that's what we buy. Because *we* buy them, food manufacturers make them. Once the big food companies figured out that they can fine tune the taste to make you buy more and more, things really got going!

Today, we eat foods that that are made, produced, and manufactured instead of merely grown, raised, and prepared; food manufacturers have made them tastier and tastier over time, because that's what 'we' demand!

We're often told to listen to our instincts, but today our instincts are failing us. We are hoarding easy calories for a famine that's never going to come. We are solving a problem that doesn't need solving, and in the process, creating a whole new series of problems.

Make no mistake; it's all us. It's all our doing, but we can also make it right.

Species-specific

We are not the only ones with instincts. Animals also have instincts. Our planet is filled with an uncountable number of animal species, and each has its *own* instincts based on driving the behaviors designed to keep it alive and thriving.

In the wild, unless some natural disaster – or worse, mankind – has messed up the environment, animals thrive on instinct alone. They eat, sleep, mate, and raise their young to do the same. Success!

Animals in zoos? Not so lucky. Pets? Yes, I'm sure they feel lucky to have *you* as an owner, but that doesn't mean they are doing as well as they could be. There is a key difference between animals in the wild, and the animals in zoos, on farms, our pets, and 99% of humanity – Animals in the wild eat the foods they are supposed to eat, and the rest of us do not.

There's a growing trend in the pet world to feed our animal loved ones the foods that they are meant to eat. In the case of cats, which are carnivores, the goal is to get them to eat mostly meat, and raw meat at that. Dogs are more omnivorous, but most modern day vets and pet owners are coming to realize that dogs aren't meant to eat processed food made of corn, wheat, and soy; 'dogs' in the wild eat meat and vegetation, not grains and legumes.

Animals can suffer from some of the same diseases of lifestyle that we can. My friend Lisa Wolfe, at Pasadena's Miracle Fitness, has a wonderful, playful dog, named Annie. Annie is fairly old, and had long suffered from the arthritis of 'age,' like so many humans do; and for years, Annie wasn't playful at all. After Lisa replaced Annie's 'healthy,' high-end commercial dog food diet with one that eliminated grains, weird byproducts, and fillers, suddenly Annie runs around and plays like dogs years younger.

Do we love our animals more than we love ourselves?

If you spend any time on Facebook, you have undoubtedly noticed that people love to share *everything* about their pets. People love animals, and they love their pets, and I don't blame them, but aside from dressing them up in little outfits and treating them as well as children, how far does it go?

The other day, we were at a high-end boutique grocery store, and try as we might, we couldn't find foods that weren't processed, boxed, and filled with questionable ingredients. Not only that, but the produce was poor quality, and the 'natural food section' wasn't natural at all.

As we were checking out, I spied a rack of gourmet canned goods; things like venison chili and bison stew. I walked over to the shelf, where I read the sign that said all the right things; all natural, organic, humanely raised, and more. Even better, the ingredients lists were *perfect*, not a bad ingredient in them.

It was dog food.

The dog food in this high-end store *for people* was better quality than anything I'd seen while specifically looking for healthy people food.

Yep, we love our pets, so we love to feed them right. What does that say about how we love ourselves?

Gorillas in the midst

...of heart attacks!

Zookeepers are now finding that animals thrive when fed the foods that their wild counterparts are eating instead of industrialized animal foods, which coincidentally are often produced by the very same manufacturers that produce mass-market pet foods.

My writer/blogger friend, John Durant (hunter-gatherer.com) turned me on to this great story, which I found particularly telling...

In 2005, a 21-year-old gorilla died of heart failure (heart disease is the number one cause of death for captive male gorillas, by the way), and prompted researchers to reexamine the lifestyles and diets of the gorillas in our nation's zoos.

At the Cleveland Zoo, they started feeding the gorillas "food such as romaine lettuce, dandelion greens, endives, alfalfa, green beans, flax seeds, and even tree branches which they strip of bark and leaves. To top it off, they give the gorillas three Centrum Silver multivitamins inside half a banana," writes David A Gabel, reporter for Environmental News Network.

As a result, the gorillas are eating more food *and* more calories, yet they are slimming down and starting to look more like their wild brothers and sisters.

"We're just recognizing that surviving on a diet and being healthy on a diet are different. We've raised our standards and are asking, are they in the best condition to not only survive but to thrive?" says Kristen Lukas, adjunct assistant professor of biology, Case Western Reserve, chair of the Gorilla Species Survival Plan®.

For this story and a great video, see the original article at enn.com/wildlife/article/42383

'I'm not an animal, I'm a human being.'

I know, you're not an animal; you're much more evolved, and you have free will. You have the choice to eat as you want, while our domesticated and captive animals only eat what we provide them. As you can see by the dog and gorilla stories, above, when we provide animals their 'species-specific diets,' they thrive. When we don't, they don't.

Dogs and cats love their treats, just like we love ours, and if they had free will (plus opposable thumbs and money), they might rebel like your teenager and buy their own junk food (just to spite you, also like your teenage daughter). Your dog, eating his unhealthy treats, would continue to live a life full of aches and pains, and be overweight and diabetic, because, as an animal, he doesn't know any better, ...but shouldn't you?

YOU on a [human] DIET

Earlier, we talked about what the wild versions of our pet dogs and cats would eat naturally, and thus stay healthy. We also showed how gorillas get healthier when given the diet that they would find in nature. Shouldn't we, mankind, also eat a diet as close to our natural diet as possible? But what is the natural human diet? What is the best diet for YOU? Your species-specific diet, of course, and your specific species is Homo sapiens.

We Homo sapiens have been around for a long time, and we are adapted best to a diet that's been around just as long.

Old Foods

The following foods are foods that most of us are well adapted to, simply because humans have been exposed to them, have eaten them, and have adapted to them for thousands of years.

- **Protein** – Meat, poultry, eggs, fish, and shellfish.

- **Vegetables** – Leaves, roots, stalks, tubers, and things like tomatoes and squash, etc.

- **Fats** – Fat from animals, foods like avocado and coconut, plus whole nuts and seeds.

- **Fruits** – By fruits I mean the sweet fruits, such as berries, stone fruits, etc., not the ones that are technically fruits but are eaten more like vegetables (think tomato). I don't want to debate fruit vs. vegetable, because that's not really the point. ...but keep your tomato out of my fruit salad!

Today's food – Many smart people have pointed out that today's foods are not the same as yesterday's. Today's fruit is bigger and sweeter, carrots are longer and more tender, and our meat isn't even the same animal, nor is it fed what *it* should be eating.

This is all true, but whether the individual food is unchanged, has disappeared, or has morphed into something almost unrecognizable, much of its underlying characteristics are still there. Plus, it's really the best we can do with what we have. We can't let perfection be the enemy of our progress.

Besides, we're not trying to live in the past; we look to the past for clues about optimal diet and health.

New foods

"You cannot assume that because we never consumed a food that we aren't adapted to it." – Mat Lalonde, Phd

I don't use Mat Lalonde's quote because I want you to eat these newer foods, but because I want to be honest with you. There are people who can eat what many paleo dieters refer to as 'Neolithic' foods and do just fine. ...or *think* they do just fine, but that's another rant, entirely.

To tell you that you aren't adapted to eat newer foods, just because ancient man didn't have access to them, would be incorrect. Dairy is a good example; many people are fully able to digest dairy, but many others are lactose intolerant or intolerant to casein (a milk protein). Dairy is a relatively new food to us, because it takes herding, shelter, and domesticated animals to produce enough milk to use as food.

Dairy is one relatively modern food that isn't all that bad. In fact, it can be very good, as long as you aren't one of the unlucky people to have intolerances to it.

The potato is another interesting food that most of us have adapted to very well, despite the newness. While the sweet potato has been around forever, white potatoes are recent in the grand scheme of things. Yet because white potatoes are mostly starch (something that healthy people can tolerate well) and low in toxins, most people handle them just fine.

In the case of the potato, it's what we do to them that's more the problem than the food itself, and the sweet potato isn't the magical tuber that health fanatics make it out to be; If the world switched to Fully Loaded Sweet Potato Skins and ate baskets of sweet potato fries every day, they would become just as demonized as the white potato, and we'd be just as fat and sick.

Hi, you must be new around here...

It's not that old is good and new is bad; the line between old and new blurs, anyway. Chili peppers are very old to the planet, but new to the Old World, since they came from the New World. That's confusing, but in this case, what's old *is* new!

Tomatoes are an even stranger story, since they have been around for a long time, but have only been eaten in large quantities since the days when Columbus took them back to Europe; they became popular, and were later re-introduced as a food to America! Even though tomatoes are 'old,' they might be new to you (intolerance to tomatoes is actually fairly common).

The foods below are just some of the foods that are most likely to have negative effects on our health. Most of them are newer to us, but like dairy and tomatoes show, it's not always time that makes it good or bad.

• **Grains & legumes** – Grains and legumes have been around for a pretty long time, but that doesn't mean we are adapted to them yet (if ever). It's only been a few thousand years since grains and legumes have been eaten in any significant quantities. You might think corn grew wild in those big yellow ears, but years ago, they were small, starchy kernels, and not sweet at all.

Grains also make tasty foods, I must admit, plus they are very cheap, making them very attractive to the budget conscious. Unfortunately, they have some less than healthful properties that can outweigh the savings. Grains and legumes are seeds of a plant, and are equipped with the protection necessary to survive to sprout and carry on the family tree; lectins, phytates, and enzyme inhibitors are all there to keep the little seed from being digested, and as a result, they can cause gut irritation and even bind to nutrients so you don't absorb them.

In addition, many popular grains, like wheat, rye, and spelt, contain a protein called gluten, which can dramatically affect the health of people who are intolerant or have celiac disease.

Traditionally, most grains and legumes were soaked, sprouted, and/or fermented before being cooked and eaten. These traditional processes removed many of the toxins that are present and tend to cause gut irritation and nutrient deficiencies.

In recent centuries, modern tools and machinery have allowed us to eat very large quantities of grains and legumes, as prices are kept artificially low by government subsidies.

Grains and legumes might be cheap calories, but from a nutrition density standpoint, they are also a poor choice. Calorie per calorie, meat, veggies, and fruit win the nutrition battle, hands down.

• **Vegetable oils** – Vegetable oils are typically high in omega-6 polyunsaturated fats, which is a fat that causes many health issues when eaten in large amounts. Polyunsatured fats are highly unstable, and oxidize quickly and easily, which many people believe leads to inflammation, particularly when consumed outside of natural sources, such as whole nuts and seeds and animal products.

For most people, there's no immediately noticeable effect of consuming vegetable oils, but trust us that the damage is being done when you don't minimize or avoid these oils.

• **Dairy** – We talked about dairy a bit earlier. Many people do fine with dairy, but a significant number of people have issues with dairy. Reports of acne, runny nose, and watery eyes are fairly common, as are the more obvious effects of lactose intolerance – gas!

Ancient diets, reimagined

Recently, we've seen some popular diets based on what our ancient ancestors ate. More likely, what we *assume* they ate; it's hard to know. Hey, judging by my local Renaissance Faire, knights and princesses were eating turkey legs, ice cream, and light beer back in the day. Going back further, to biblical times or the times of the 'caveman' is even more problematic!

Paleo Diet – This diet looks to how our ancient, ancient, ancient ancestors might have eaten, and takes dietary cues from their history. We don't need to eat what they ate to have success. We look at how they ate for clues on to what to eat to thrive, instead of just survive. Most Paleo diets start off pretty strict and allow you to reintroduce *some* foods to test how you feel. Things like veggies, meat, fruit, and eggs are in, while things like grains, legumes, sugars, and dairy tend to be out!

Primal –This version of the Paleo Diet was popularized by Mark Sisson, author of *The Primal Blueprint,* although in some ways it's a tomato vs. *tomahto* thing compared to Paleo. Mark's version is more approachable to many, primarily because it doesn't start off quite as strict. It's also known for being more cool with some dairy. …assuming it's not a problem.

Biblically based diets – The *Maker's Diet* and *What Would Jesus Eat* are attempts to eat more like our biblical ancestors, which meant fewer grains and legumes and more vegetables, meat, fish, and fruit.

'Real Food' – The "30 Days of Real Food" & *The Real Food Reset* have a lot in common with these other diets. Ours starts with the premise that people who eat closer to how humans are meant to eat, tend to do better, just like our pets and zoo animals do on their natural diets.

We are an adaptive species

We're not exactly the same as we were thousands of years ago, but we also haven't changed all that much in the grand scheme of things. We vary in our abilities to handle certain foods based on where our ancestors came from and what they ate for generations. Even with those differences, our primary sources of nutrition will tend to be very similar, even if some of us can thrive on variations in ingredients, amounts, and ratios.

Good decisions, bad decisions

If there's a major downside to being human, it's our consciousness. I'm not trying to be deep or especially profound, but this is becoming a problem.

As people, we think. We're self-aware. We make decisions. And we make bad ones, quite often.

You see, just because we are self-aware, doesn't make us aware of when our instincts are leading us astray – something they can often do.

We live in a modern world that's so far removed from our natural, ancestral environment that our instincts are confused. Our instincts were designed to keep us alive in a world where beasts and monsters are around every corner, and food is hard to hunt and kill OR time consuming to gather.

In our instinctive world, it pays off to have a thin[nish] layer of fat on your body, just in case you can't find shelter tonight or food for breakfast when you wake up. Today, though, modern food what it is, it's hard to stop at just a thin layer of fat on our bodies. Not that we ever need that thin layer today, anyway, right?

Yes, in the past, the prospect of starvation was always looming over us, and our instincts prepared us for the worst. In a modern world where the worst case scenario tends to be oversleeping and leaving the house hungry, our instincts are a little too powerful. In fact, when truly bad things are *unlikely* to happen, and modern industrialized foods are cheap and plentiful, we get fat and sick, instead.

Survive, yes. Thrive, no.

Fat, sick, and ready to believe it's inevitable

I use the word 'fat' in the heading because it's easy to understand. Many of us *are* fat; in fact I was fat for 35 of my 45 years before I got my act together.

Yes, we understand 'fat' because we see it every day, whether it's in our family, friends, or in the mirror, but what we tend to overlook is the fraternal twin brother of being fat, which is being sick.

Most of us know *someone* with one or more of the following diseases or conditions:

- Diabetes (Type 2)
- Metabolic Syndrome
- Arthritis

- Thyroid Disease
- Depression
- Celiac Disease
- Chronic Constipation
- Heartburn or GERD
- Heart Disease
- High Cholesterol
- High Blood Pressure

While we all know people with one or more of these diseases, we seem to take them in stride, almost as if they are inevitable. It's sad that most people consider these things to be normal these days, but is it normal or simply typical?

Normal vs Typical vs Natural

Many people call today's human conditions 'normal,' but that doesn't tell the whole story.

- My friend Katy Bowman, MS, the brain behind the Restorative Exercise™ Institute says that what's normal today certainly isn't natural, but over time, things have changed. These changes happened slowly, and for the most part, went unnoticed. ...until now.

- Paul Chek, a popular, if controversial, Holistic Health Coach, says that we've become accustomed to the feeling of being 'sick,' and no longer feel it's a problem; it's all we know.

What's normal today wasn't normal just a few years ago, much less for our ancient ancestors. Today, we pay the price, often without knowing it.

The new normal

I like to call our modern condition (which is often sick and overweight) the 'new normal,' even though they aren't really all that new anymore, and they certainly aren't normal, much less natural.

The Centers for Disease Control reported in 2012 that over 69% of Americans are overweight, over 38% are obese, and over 8% have type 2 diabetes. While these numbers are the highest they've ever been, make no mistake, they've been high for a long time, and have gotten higher every year.

With these numbers, the odds are good that one or more of these conditions personally affects you or someone close to you. It's no wonder we hardly raise an eyebrow. We see it, on a personal level, almost every day!

Like father like son

Doctors and insurance companies like to get your family history, and news reports often talk about how your odds increase or decrease based on whether someone in your immediate family has the condition.

Yes, you can argue that many of these conditions have a genetic component to them, and it's true; certain people are more likely to contract these conditions, based on their genes. But, we can't discount the cultural element of the family history principle, either. If your parents' lifestyle helped to bring on the condition, odds are you are living a similar lifestyle, since you tend to learn from your parents.

In most cases, genetics only make you more susceptible to a condition, and don't guarantee you'll develop it; just like a family history that's free and clear doesn't mean you're risk free. To a large degree, what you do to your body can trigger disease as much, or more so, than pure genetics. If one has a family history of Type 2 Diabetes or carries the 'celiac gene,' they are much more likely to exhibit symptoms and suffer the effects of the disease if they live (and eat) the lifestyle that's going to set it off. In celiac, it's primarily wheat and other gluten containing grains that trigger the detrimental effects, although a high stress lifestyle, a lack of sleep, and an otherwise poor diet can push things over the edge. In Type 2 Diabetes, it's a diet too high in carbohydrate and a lack of activity – over many years – that are the most obvious triggers. Today, we're seeing that people with lifestyles high in stress and highly inflammatory foods can make things worse OR trigger Type 2 *years* before a sedentary or high carb diet, alone, might.

Overriding your instincts

We love to use the term 'animal instincts' to talk about those times when we just let things take over. When we let our emotions take over, and we seem out of control: sexual urges, running in fear, or turning to fight are some of the animal instincts that we feel on a regular basis. Those urges seem pretty positive, as long as they are acted on appropriately.

There's also a flip side to our animal nature, and when it takes over, we can give into that urge to eat things that just aren't good for us, or to overeat foods that might otherwise be good, if only eaten in smaller, more appropriate quantities. These are animal urges, too.

But we're not animals, are we? We're smart enough to push those out of place instincts aside, and rely on our brains and experience. We are smart enough to see that our instincts are failing us, and educated enough to see what it's leading to. We are ready to turn this ship around.

"Be a good animal, true to your animal instincts." – DH Lawrence

The Real Food Reset

In the previous chapters, we gave you a little bit of dietary history, and debunked the idea of the detox or cleanse. There's no 'magic pill' to get your insides healthy, whether it comes in the form of a supplement, a juice blend, green smoothies, or an enema bag. What IS the key, is eating real food, which maximizes the good food, minimizes the bad, and creates healthy habits.

There are many ways to transition to a real food diet – you can slowly start to wean yourself off of packaged foods, read labels more carefully, and stop having your afternoon mochaccino. You can even buy one of those popular diet books that have all the menus and supplements figured out for you, so you can just follow a plan. We are not saying that won't work, but it may take a while to do all of that.

How much longer are you willing to go on with less than your usual energy? Extra rolls of fat on your belly? Digestive distress? Depression? Acne? Have you ever wondered if there wasn't something you could do with nutrition? There is, but you have to take a smart and proven approach.

We created our 30 Day Reset with one goal, which is to take you from where you are now to where you deserve to be, in just one month.

Unlike a diet, a reset actually works with the natural program of your body – it won't starve you, make you tired, or stress you out. On the contrary – it will free your physical, emotional and mental potential and it will teach you valuable lessons and habits on the way!

It really works!

Here's the reason why resets work; by feeding your body real food and allowing yourself enough movement and rest, you clean up the 'bugs' in your system and optimize your body's software. Cells get new information and are able to grow and divide using healthy building blocks, your digestion is running smoothly, your brain is sharp, your muscle tissue grows, your skin is brighter, your hair and nails look healthier, your mood is better, your social life is bubbling again. In a nutshell, your quality of life improves. We have plenty of scientific data to believe that even 3 weeks of eating real food allows your genes to turn off the fat storage mode and make you into a healthy lean beast if you just keep on going! Just by eating real food and moving some? You bet!

The goal of a reset

The goal of a reset is to allow your body to work optimally, but also to remind you to take better care of yourself, to be able to control the controllables in your life and to manage the factors that you cannot control with more ease.

After these first '30 days,' you will enjoy a new mindset, a rekindled relationship with food and its origins, a better understanding of when you are full or hungry, and some of you will have beat serious sugar, savory snack, or grain addiction.

Get your mind on board

How often have you started a plan only to abandon it 3 days later? Most people blame themselves for lack of willpower, but we have found that the main reason most of us fail is because we expect to feed our body the right food but we forget to feed our mind first.

What was that expression: "mind over matter?" You cannot take your body anywhere without your mind going in the same direction. In fact, expect that in order for your body to transform naturally, you need your mind to be leading the way. If you have not been training your mind, you have been missing out on a great opportunity, so let's start now.

1. In your imagination, draw a picture, or even make a movie, of where you want to be in 30 days. Imagine how you look and feel, the things you are able to do, the obstacles that are lifted! What does that look like or feel like? Maybe it's something like: "I am lighter, I have energy to do my work, I am having fun cooking with my wife," or "My hands feel free of pain, I work with joy! I am gardening every day!"

2. Write your statement on a piece of paper and place it somewhere visible – on your nightstand, desk, or the

fridge door. Repeat it to yourself a number of times in the present tense, say: "In 30 days I am lighter, energetic and healthier!"

3. Involve others. Have them say that statement back to you. Ask your wife or friend or colleague to say the same to you: "In 30 days you are lighter, energetic and healthier!" Hearing it from someone else makes your mind desire *achieving* that goal, so eating the way that will get you there comes with less effort. You can make that statement as customized and specific as you like.

"I am starting my 30 days of real food reset. In 30 days I am… _____." Fill in the blanks.

Make sure you read that statement at least twice a day – Changing your mind won't happen without your participation.

Won't it be fantastic when one month from now someone asks you why you look so different, and you get to say:

"It wasn't hard at all – I ate real food and paid attention to my thoughts twice a day!"

Read on and see how our promise is different from anything else you've tried before.

The empty promise

…that really only leads to empty bowels.

Health claims aside, most of the products or plans that you are likely to come across on the internet have common themes:

- They tell you that "you don't have it in you," and by giving you a simple, sparse, and Spartan regimen to follow, they take a lot of your choices away.

- By giving you a short timeframe, they hope you'll be able to stick it out.

- By making sketchy promises of health and/or weight loss success based on little, misrepresented, or NO science, they give you the hope that they know you need to keep on track for _____ # of days.

I know, our plan also has a timeframe, but it's not that short. It's also not that the expected drab, boring diet of chicken breast and broccoli, which should make the time pass more quickly. We're also not promising you anything magical, we won't tell you that you will lose 15 lbs. in 7 days, and we won't tell you that our plan will make you look 10 years younger by next week. You should feel much better, and our plan will help you stay that way. If you feel more energetic, you will stay that way, too. If you follow our plan and lose 10 lbs., you will maintain that weight loss when you are done, and you will walk away with lasting health, improved performance, and a feeling of well-being.

We've called our plan "the 30 Days of Real Food" or "The Real Food Reset" for some time now, and since we've being running 'resets' with clients and friends, we've found that they really do seem to 'reset' people and their relationship with food.

The big button reset

A reset works very much like that big button on your computer. When your mouse freezes, when a program doesn't work, when you are frustrated with how slowly something is going, or when you just don't know why your computer is 'stuck,' you press the big button. The start screen appears, you type in your password and oh, a miracle, everything works. We humans get stuck the same way a computer gets stuck, and the way to unstick ourselves is to go back to our more natural state of eating and moving like we are designed to.

I won't take too much time to explain this, but let's just say 100 years ago we didn't have the foods we have today, and 10,000 years ago we had even fewer of them. We have not had adequate time to adapt to a lot of these new foods, and sometimes eating a bit too much of them may just be too stressful for our poor bodies to handle. If we pay attention, we might find that we've had too much of our modern foods by displaying some of the following signs: fatigue, trouble sleeping, digestive distress, lack of energy, poor performance, brain fog, allergies, obsessive thoughts of food and overeating at night, anxiety, depression, aggression, hormonal imbalances, lack of sex drive, lack of motivation, etc.

Just like you would press the big button on your computer to make your programs run well again, you can apply the same trick to your own body and reset it by eating the right foods and adding a bit more movement into your life.

It's all about the [real] food

We could drone on and on about the nutrition, building a case for quality protein sources, nutrient rich carbohydrates, and healthy fats, but the bottom line is that a diet of 'real food' is going to limit some foods and highlight some others.

Many of the foods that we've grown up with simply aren't all that healthy, particularly in the amounts that our collective culture has come to enjoy. Our species grew up eating meat, eggs, veggies, fruit, nuts and seeds, and the base of our food pyramid was never based on grains and carbohydrates until our governments and their departments of agriculture got involved.

I don't want to get too political, so I'll keep this short and sweet, and let government conspiracy experts handle the rants; I believe that many people in the government *do* care about your health, but they also care about farmers, ranchers, doctors, and dentists. Unfortunately, it seems that the mouthpieces of the farmers, ranchers, doctors, and dentist have become 'represented' by big corporate and big government mouthpieces, and not the traditional people that you'd expect. This means that they are heavily influenced by the very politics that I don't like to get into.

It's not that I'm putting my fingers in my ears and pretending not to listen, I just don't have it in me to rant, while others do a much better job. In the resources section (EatMoveLive52.com/30Days), we have a few links to websites that rant much better than we ever will!

Ok, time to get back on track; less food policy, and more food itself!

Good Guys (eat these)

We'll get to details in the next few pages, but here's a short list of the foods that are best for us, and should be the base of your 'real food' diet for the next 30 days.

Protein – beef, pork, chicken, fish, shellfish, eggs, game meats, other poultry, and even sources of protein like bacon, sausage, bison, and venison are fair game (pun intended).

Vegetables – green leafy vegetables, broccoli, avocado, cauliflower, Brussels sprouts, cabbage, artichokes, green beans, snow peas, sugar snap peas, asparagus, zucchini, squash, eggplant, tomatoes, peppers, onion, garlic, leeks, shallots, beets, golden beets, beet greens and other greens, kale, carrots, parsnips, jicama, radishes, mushrooms, etc. Yes, we know some of these are technically fruits and fungus...

Protein and vegetables should be the true base of your 'Real Food Reset.' Yes, you will have other foods, but these two items should be your primary focus.

Healthy Fats – avocado, olive oil, lard, coconut oil, butter, ghee, bacon fat, coconut milk, olives, etc.

Fats are healthy and necessary, but until you get good at this 'real food thing,' don't worry so much about *adding* fats. Rest assured that you are getting plenty of fats from meats and other protein sources, foods like avocado, and some added fat for cooking, when necessary. That being said, some fats are better for you than others, and we will show you the best ones in the next chapter

Fruit – We generally suggest people start with one serving of whole fruit per day.

Nuts & seeds – We suggest that nuts and seeds make great condiments, so-so snacks, and *terrible* foods to have as daily staples. They are simply too delicious and calorie rich. You MUST control yourself, and keep it to a serving a day. If you can't do that, skip the nuts, at least for the first 30 days.

Dairy – Like nuts, dairy is delicious, and can be high in calories. In addition, for many people dairy simply doesn't register as food, and they can easily overeat it. Also, dairy is one of the foods that many people have issues with, even if they don't know it. Consider going 30 days without it, then trying it again.

Fruit, nuts, seeds, and dairy aren't bad, per se, but they shouldn't be foods to focus on. They are condiments, side dishes, snacks, desserts, and ingredients to be added to real meals, not the basis of meals in and of themselves.

Bad Guys (don't eat these)

We covered the 'good guys' above, so here comes the painful part; the list of the foods that aren't as good for us, and should be minimized in general, but *specifically* minimized for the first 30 days of your 'Real Food Reset.'

I will remind you that our goal is to have you eliminate these foods for the first 30 days of your 'Reset,' after which you can choose to reintroduce foods if you wish. We're not saying this list of foods is evil or horrible for everyone, but these foods are implicated in many metabolic and health issues, like obesity, auto-immune conditions, gut and bowel problems, and more.

Go 30 days without, and then let us show you how to reintroduce some of them to see how you feel.

Grains and grain products – wheat, oats, rye, barley, rice, corn, wild rice, plus things made from them, like bread, cakes, cookies, tortillas, chips, corn meal, corn bread, oatmeal, couscous, pasta, noodles, etc.

"There are millions of people and dozens of cultures around the world who do just fine with grains in their diets." – the many scientists, nutritionists, dieticians, and other people who really want to eat donuts.

While I have to agree with the quote, I do have several responses:

- Most of these cultures also live lives with more activity, more sleep, less stress, otherwise healthy diets. Things add up, and when everything else is good, your poor dietary choices don't matter as much.

- Many of these cultures eat very little food in general, and under calorie restriction, they also eat a very low amount of 'bad foods.' Under these positive circumstances, the bad foods that they do eat seem to have a negligible effect on health.

- How much better would they be doing if they actually *removed* grains from their diets?

Even if grains aren't evil, they simply aren't necessary. Not by a long shot. Calorie per calorie, they hold little in the way of nutrition compared to vegetables, meat, and most fruit.

"Millions of people and many cultures around the world do just fine, if not even better, without grains in their diets." – Roland Denzel

This quote is also true, and I'll hazard a guess that a comparison between the two types of populations would show that those without grains tend to be healthier and have reduced rates of 'age and lifestyle related illnesses.'

Grain-like seeds and seed products – quinoa, buckwheat, amaranth, etc.

These faux grains are technically not grains at all, but they might as well be the same thing. They have similar properties and nutritional profiles. In the amounts that most of us eat today, they aren't much of an issue, but if you were to replace all of your grain based foods with these food sources, you'd likely be in the same boat.

Legumes and legume products – soybeans, peanuts, beans, lentils, chickpeas, peas, hummus, etc.

Like whole grains, legumes have a mystique of healthfulness. We'll admit that they are better than most grains, but nutritionally, they still pale in comparison to meats, fish, veggies, etc.

Trans fats – partially hydrogenated oils, margarine, shortening, often found in snacks and baked treats.

These are artificially created solid fats that have been shown to cause heart disease, etc. Avoid them with a capital A.

Sugar(s) – Any sugar, no matter how brown or natural it looks. Sugar is sugar. Also, avoid molasses, honey, high fructose corn syrup, maltodextrin, fructose, dextrose, sucrose, maltose, maple syrup, agave syrup, fruit syrup or concentrate, etc.

Not all of these 'sugars' are true sugars, but they are the same thing to the body, and sugar is sugar. If you'd like to read more, see our post called "Sugar: You keep using that word" at http://eatmovelive52.com/sugarword

Artificial Sweeteners – Acesulfame K (E950), Aspartame (E951), Saccharin (E954), Sucralose (E955) are the actual names (and E numbers in Europe) for common artificial sweeteners such as Splenda, NutraSweet, Sweet N Low, etc.

Stevia – What about stevia and those other, exotic, natural sweeteners? We're trying to break the sugar habit, and sweet things will string you along even longer. **For 30**

days, stop adding things to your food and drinks that make them sweeter!

Liquids with calories – soda, pop, juice, sweetened tea and coffee, sports, drinks, fancy coffee drinks, fast food shakes, fruity smoothies, etc.

Liquid calories often don't register as 'food,' so you're likely to be just as hungry after you drink them as before, so these are wasted, empty calories, and often sugary ones at that.

Alcohol – beer, wine, and liquor.

Calories aside, alcohol causes many people to lose their inhibitions with many things, food choices included. In addition, because alcohol registers with the body as 'toxic,' it must be preferentially processed by the body to eliminate it. During that time, you've effectively shut off any fat burning and produced byproducts that are easily stored as fat. Alcohol also makes sleep worse, not better. All of these things leave you more susceptible to making bad choices.

'Bad' Fats – Corn oil, Soybean oil, most prepared salad dressings, vegetable oil, sunflower oil, safflower oil, margarines, shortening, hydrogenated fats, trans fats, non-dairy creamers, etc.

These fats are rich in omega-6 fatty acids, which are necessary to the body, in moderation. The modern industrialized diet contains up to 10-20 times the amounts that are needed and healthy, and as a result leaves us in a state of systemic inflammation because of the imbalance.

Avoid these fats, which so are cheap and plentiful that they seem to be in everything.

Packaged and processed foods – Most processed foods, packaged foods, restaurant foods, and fast foods (but not all) contain many of the above ingredients. If you're not sure, skip them.

Fast foods and other restaurant foods are often breaded, fried in poor quality 'bad' fats, and more bun than burger.

While you can get a decent meal when you're out and about, you must be careful, do your research, and think before you eat. When in doubt, pass them up, and eat at home whenever possible, at least during your first 30 days.

Let's do this!

As with every adventure, you can't just start. You need to spend some time preparing in order to be successful in your reset. Luckily, it's very simple to prepare for the 30 days of *The Real Food Reset*.

First, get out a piece of paper, or download and print out the form in our "30 Days Food List," found at EatMoveLive52.com/30Days.

Second, look at the list below and write down (or circle on your printed form) all the foods you would enjoy eating during the next 30 days. Imagine yourself buying, cooking, ordering, and tasting them, clearly picture yourself with a plate of those foods in front of you – this will help you choose the foods you need to stock in your fridge and pantry, as the ones that are most important to you are going to stand out.

To make it easy we have listed all 'great for you foods' first, and we'll cover the ones you should stay away from later. After the 'bad guys,' we will also show you some foods that you may want to consider eliminating if you have certain allergies or suspect intolerances.

Focus on these foods

Protein – and vegetables, of course – are the core of *The Real Food Reset*, and since most meals focus on either the meat or the veggie, we've started with those two categories so it's easier to plan and visualize your meals. The following 'great for you foods' should be the focus during your 30 Day Real Food Reset.

Protein Sources

Protein sources are typically things like beef, pork, chicken, fish, and shellfish, but also include eggs and some dairy.

As you read the list, below, you might notice that we do not specify 'lean meats' or tell you to trim the fat before cooking. Fat is an essential part of the human diet, and animal fat has been incorrectly demonized over the years. We've seen that the government's policies to limit animal fats, and even fats in general, haven't had the desired effect of reducing heart disease, but we have long been told that 'no studies existed' that proved these policies to be wrong. Without evidence, the policies continued; foods like butter and lard were guilty until proven innocent.

Actually, butter might be more than just *not guilty*, butter might be truly innocent. The crime *might* be that butter hasn't been allowed to help, all these years.

In 2012, data was 'unearthed' that showed that waaaaaay back in the '60s and '70s, there were studies to test whether seed oils were healthier than animal fats, and therefore better for the heart (*BMJ 2013;346:e8707*). It turns out that merely swapping safflower oil products for animal fat products **increased** coronary heart disease related deaths by 61% (16.3% vs. 10.1%) cardiovascular

related deaths by 56% (17.2% vs. 11%), and all-cause
mortality by 49% (17.6% vs. 11.8%).

We still don't know what happened to these studies
way back when, and why the data was misplaced, lost,
ignored, or forgotten, but it's a shame that they are only
being looked at now. It looks like we've been following
very bad advice for many years, and watched our country's
heart disease numbers rise, rather than fall.

Thankfully, many doctors and dieticians are coming
around to the healthfulness of natural fats, so go ahead
and experiment with the cuts of meat (and even whole
eggs, butter, and lard) that you love, whether they are
lean or fatty. Animal fat has been demonized far too long.

Beef (any type or cut)
Pork (any type or cut)
Lamb (any type or cut)
Game and other meats (any type or cut)
Chicken (any type or cut)
Turkey (any type or cut)
Game birds and other fowl (any type or cut)
Bacon & sausage (yes, we know they are made of meat,
but people always ask)
Fish and shellfish
Whole eggs
Protein powders (whey, casein, milk, egg, etc.)
Cottage cheese
Greek yogurt

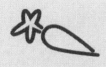

But wait, I'm a vegetarian!

...and I can't eat some of the protein sources you suggest!

We understand and respect your choice to not eat meat.

To get adequate protein, focus on eggs, dairy, and legumes. You can also purchase rice, pea and hemp protein powders to prepare shakes.

For a lot of vegetarians, the 'do not eat' list is even more important. Focus on avoiding the foods that you should NOT eat, and do your best with the rest!

Vegetables

Most vegetables are high in nutrition per calorie, and are virtually unlimited. If you're the type to binge on squash, for instance, then you'll have to limit them. For this reason, we've moved some higher calorie vegetables, such as sweet potatoes and yams, to another category to make things easier to manage. More on this, later.

Green leafy vegetables (lettuce, spinach, kale, etc.)
Broccoli
Cauliflower
Brussels sprouts
Cabbage
Artichokes
Green beans, snow peas, sugar snap peas (technically legumes, but more pod than pea)
Asparagus

Zucchini
Summer squash
Squash
Eggplant
Tomato
Pepper
Onion and green onion
Garlic, leeks, shallots
Beets, golden beets, beet greens
Carrots
Jicama
Radish
Mushrooms
**Fermented vegetables (kim chi, sauerkraut, pickles, other
pickled veggies)**

Fats

Fat is already in many of the foods that we eat from
the lists, above. Meat, eggs, poultry, and fish all contain fat
already, so unless you choose to eat only very lean protein
sources, you're getting enough fat, even before *adding* fat.

For cooking, butter and liquid fats from this list can be
used, and if you need oil for a salad dressing, choose olive
oil.

Coconut milk, which is concentrated coconut, not the
one that's marketed as a milk replacement, can be used to
flavor soups, stews, and curries, or used instead of cream
in coffee (an acquired taste). Most good coconut milk is
very thick, and sold in cans or jars, not 'milk cartons.'

Healthy or not, it is still very high in calories and can be overeaten. Use it in moderation.

The additional items (bacon, avocado, olives, and nuts) are great sources of fat that can be used as condiments and flavor enhancers, but should not be used a primary source of protein or vegetable during your 30 days of *The Real Food Reset.*

Butter or ghee
Bacon fat
Coconut oil
Olive oil (any 100% olive oil variety)
Coconut milk (not the 'milk carton' variety)
Bacon
Avocado
Olives
Nuts (shelled yourself, whenever possible)

Drinks

You can have unlimited calorie free drinks from the following list.

Water
Sparkling water
Unsweetened ice tea
Kombucha (plain and unsweetened)
Tea and coffee (black or with cream/milk/butter) *

* If the drink has calories (from cream, etc.) then it should be limited to 1-2 servings per day. Drinks like

kombucha and bottled teas can vary wildly in calories, so if it has more than 5-10 per serving, look out for added sweeteners. Remember, one goal is to break the sugar habit, and sweet drinks just drag things out

Fruits

1-2 servings per day. Yes, fruit has all sorts of healthful properties, but fruit is also overrated compared to veggies. Higher in calories, and often high in sugar, fruits are not something that should be eaten in large amounts. Some fruits are sugar bombs, and have to be even more restricted, especially during a fat loss phase. Also, some fruits are simply too big to be just one serving (think of a large banana or a big apple, which are closer to two servings). Make sure that you follow the spirit of the plan, and don't try to exploit the loopholes; you only have yourself to exploit. See 'Direct Carbohydrate,' below, for more information...

Berries (fresh or frozen)
Papaya
Pineapple
Pomegranate
Apple
Citrus fruit
Lemon
Lime
Limited amounts of other fruits

What about faux food

When people start to diet, some foods are off limits! When foods go 'off limits,' fake food versions start to appear on store shelves!

As we learned during the 'low fat' craze of the 90s, foods that replace one bad ingredient with another can be just as bad, and just as fattening (hello, Snack Wells!).

During the 30 days of 'Real Food,' avoid foods that are designed to mimic the foods that you are trying to minimize or eliminate; this means steering clear of pastas, cakes, cookies, drinks, and other foods, even if they claim to be gluten free, low carb, sugar free, or 'paleo.'

This 30 days is as much about resetting our food attitudes as it is about resetting our digestive systems!

Herbs, spices, condiments

Herbs and spices are almost always calorie free or so low in calories that it just doesn't matter. Use them all you like.

Sea salt and Himalayan salt
Fresh herbs, dried spices and natural spice mixes
Mustard (beware sauces filled with 'bad guys')
Horseradish (beware sauces filled with 'bad guys')
Fresh lemon juice
Vinegar

Beware of jarred and bottled sauces and condiments, as they can be full of things you wouldn't expect, and condensed down so that a mere tablespoon can have as many calories as a dessert topping or salad dressing.

Direct carbohydrate

It's really hard to give a catchy name to a category filled with high-starch, high-calorie, and high-sugar foods that are otherwise natural and healthy (without sounding like an extremist). It must be done, though.

Healthy or not, we have goals for our 30 days of *The Real Food Reset*, and they include fighting off sugar addiction, quite possibly losing weight, and often dropping extra body fat. With these goals in mind, it's hard to let you go *whole hog* on 'carbs.'

Note that these foods are not strictly off limits, nor are they free to be eaten at will. They should be minimized if fat loss is a goal. If there are a few chunks of potato or turnip in your stew, don't sweat it, but for the 30 days of *The Real Food Reset*, you should only consider eating foods from this category if you exercise intensely and don't want to lose weight. Otherwise, minimize these foods. After your first 30 days, you will have the chance to reintroduce more of these foods more freely.

Sweet potatoes
Yams
Potatoes
Yucca
Parsnips

Turnips
Rutabagas
Honey (in small amounts)
Yogurt (avoid mass produced, sweetened yogurt)
Kefir (avoid mass produced, sweetened kefir)
Coconut water (in moderation)
Chocolate (yes, even *dark* chocolate)

Completely avoid these foods

Why are these foods in parenthesis? That's how negative numbers are often shown in accounting ledgers and spreadsheets to make them stand out when color isn't an option.

These 'negative' foods are foods that should be avoided, especially during your first 30 days!

(Bread, tortillas, muffins, cakes, pies, noodles, etc.)
(Grains including wheat and wheat flour, rye, barley, rice, etc.)
(Corn and other grass seeds, like wild rice, corn tortillas, chips, corn meal)
(Grain-like seeds, like quinoa, buckwheat, etc.)
(Beans, legumes, hummus, etc. (pea pods and green beans are fine))
(Oats and oatmeal)
(Pasta and noodles – corn, soba, rice, quinoa)
(Corn oil)
(Soybean oil)
(Vegetable oil)

(Seed, grain, and legume oils – sunflower, safflower, rice
bran, soybean, etc.)
(Salad dressings – because most store bought dressings
contain seed oils)
(Hydrogenated fats)
(Trans fats)
(Margarine)
(Shortening)
(Non-dairy creamer)
(Non-dairy products)
(Sugar)
(Honey)
(Artificial sweeteners)
(High fructose corn syrup)
(Sodas)
(Juices)
('Healthy,' 'sports,' and 'diet' drinks)
(Fancy coffee drinks)
(Alcohol)
(Processed, packaged foods)
(Most fast foods (see fast food guide later))
(Fried and breaded foods)
(Soy products)

Minimize these foods

It's not that these next foods are necessarily bad, but
these foods are not very satiating for many people,
contain a lot of calories, are easily overeaten and/or
stimulate appetite. Use them in moderation, as

condiments or toppings, or not at all. These foods are not to be primary sources of nutrition, especially during the first 30 days or whenever fat loss is a goal.

A sharp eye will notice that some of these foods appear on multiple lists, as your body can react differently to certain foods under different circumstances (when sedentary vs. when very active, for instance).

Direct Carbohydrates (see the Direct Carb list on previous pages)
Nuts and seeds (only eat if you shell them yourself)
Cheese
Yogurt
Stevia
Honey

You might have noticed that Greek yogurt and cottage cheese appear on the Protein Sources list, but here we urge you to minimize yogurt and cheese. Why the discrepancy? Greek yogurt and cottage cheese tend to be far more satiating than regular cheese and yogurt, being higher in protein and lower in carbohydrate. Just remember to avoid the ones that are flavored and sweetened.

Avoid these foods if you have allergies

Many of our clients, family, and friends are sniffly and sneezy, itchy and scratchy, or have a variety of conditions that seem to be affected by foods, including acne, rheumatoid arthritis, dermatitis, irritable bowel syndrome, lupus, asthma, and more. The evidence is inconclusive that food is the cause, but there's little to dispute when people seem to 'get better' during an elimination diet and 'get worse' when they add those foods back in.

If you suspect you might have 'issues,' then you owe it to yourself to go at least 30 days on a more strict elimination diet; which includes skipping the following foods, in addition to the 'do not eat' list, above.

If you suspect an allergy or intolerance, you should avoid:

You will notice that many of these items are on the recommended lists, but that doesn't mean they are good for YOU! Any foods you know or suspect to be related to an allergy or intolerance should be avoided.

Dairy
Eggs
Soy
Wheat & grains, gluten-free or not
Seeds, nuts, peanuts, legumes
Tomatoes
Peppers
Potatoes
Eggplant
Alcohol

You might be exhausted and confused from scrolling up and down to take in these lists, but it won't take too long to get familiar with what foods are the ones to focus on eating and the ones that you're going to avoid or minimize for a while.

To make things easier, we have a downloadable document on our website that you can print off to keep handy for shopping trips, or just to stick to the fridge. It's available at EatMoveLive52.com/30Days, and is called the "30 Days of Real Food Fridge Poster and Pocket Guide".

But isn't _____ a 'healthy' carb?

Foods like yogurt, kefir, dark chocolate, and coconut water are often sold as health foods, giving people the illusion that they can be eaten freely or that more is better.

These foods are the darling children of the health conscious, but just like your own darling children, they aren't right for everybody, and are sometimes better in small doses!

To make matters worse, many of these products take the health benefit of the main ingredient, and mix it will all sorts of unhealthy things, yet still claim it's healthy.

Foods like yogurt, kefir, and chocolate are good examples. In their raw and plain form, they are great for us, but in order to make them delicious for consumers, they get sweetened and flavored, which can nullify the benefits, or worse, make them *bad* for you.

Coconut water is basically little more than sugar water, no matter what the advertising says. Is it better than a sports drink? Barely...

Planning and preparing

Take your time to plan and prepare for this transition. You can download and print the 30 days food list at EatMoveLive52.com/30Days, and use it to follow along during the next step: cleaning out the kitchen, restocking it, and planning your meals.

Pantry and fridge clean up

At this point you may be finding out that your fridge and pantry are stocked with some items that are featured on our 'do not eat' list. Stay calm and focused and look through labels to determine which foods can still be a part of your diet and which need to go. Of course, you'll likely find that foods without labels and ingredient lists are far more likely to be on the recommended lists. It's funny that way, huh?

We realize there may be other people in your household who are enjoying their snacks, salad dressings, breads, and soy products, so don't make them miserable and angry by throwing their food out under the cover of night. Instead, clean up a shelf in the fridge and pantry for your own foods and, if possible, place the incompatible foods out of sight so you're not constantly tempted. If you know the peanut butter will be calling your name from the fridge, move it in a cupboard where you cannot reach, give it away, or even toss it. It's only 30 days after all.

To the store!

First take out the list of favorite, allowed foods – the one that you wrote or printed off and circled. Look at the foods that you circled, and also at the lists of recommended foods; pick proteins, fats, veggies and fruits that you enjoy. Make a shopping list, then it's off to the store. You don't need to buy a lot of these items on day 1 but plan for at least 3 days –that means 9-12 meals.

It helps to know your way around a grocery store, but since most of the foods are fresh or frozen, most will be found around the perimeter of the store – this is where most of the fresh food is.

You should buy as much of your food as you can fresh, but frozen veggies, fruits and meat are also fine. They store longer and make cooking easy. You can also pick up some cans of tuna, coconut milk, and pickled vegetables so that you can prepare good food in a hurry.

For more information on acceptable packaged and prepared foods from the store, visit Meal Survivor (mealsurvivor.com). We have reviewed many high quality items there, and barring our advice about allergies and intolerances, most are compliant with our suggestions *after* your initial 30 days of *The Real Food Reset.*

Sidebar –What about organic?

Many people get panicky when they start to diet, thinking that they need to buy all organic and expensive foods. Strangely, they often choose to stick to their diet of donuts and fast food over a healthier diet of conventionally grown veggies and protein sources.

"Don't let perfection be the enemy of progress." – Unknown

Non-organic veggies, eggs, fruit, dairy, and meat will still be better than even the most organic and 'natural' cookies, cereals, and salty snacks.

Not all produce 'is created equal,' or in this case grown equally; some fruits and vegetables have been found to be safer than others. Every year, the Environmental Working Group releases its lists of the Dirty Dozen worst offenders, and the Clean 15, which is the list of those items found to be lowest in pesticides.

Dirty Dozen & Clean 15: ewg.org/foodnews

Plan your menu

You can download a printable menu design sheet from our website (EatMoveLive52.com/30Days). Print it out or simply open it on your computer screen. It's time to get planning!

Think of your week – which days can you eat at home, which days do you just have to run out the door or eat out. Do the same drill with your lunches – will you be eating out or bringing food from home? Look at dinners and social calendars. The key here is to know what your week's schedule looks like, so you can prepare well in advance.

How many meals?

We suggest that you shoot for 3 meals with 1 small snack in between, especially if you are already physically active. 2 meals works for some people but you may tend to be hungry and overeat. Think of what works best with your schedule and appointments, but have a good breakfast, lunch and dinner on most days.

How many calories?

Your focus on the 30 days of *The Real Food Reset* is to eat real food, and trust that getting adequate nutrition will be enough to guide your appetite. For this reason, you won't be counting calories. Yeah!

How much to eat?

Serve yourself what you would consider a 'regular portion.' That may vary depending on your size, but if you are a 220 lb. male, 2 eggs won't do it for you. Make sure you eat enough food so you can go without eating for at least 4-5 hours.

How to rate satiety?

Your fullness is determined by the duration of your meal, how well you chewed, how well you paid attention to the process of eating and to the food on your plate. If you are aware in your eating and pay attention to the colors, textures, flavors and recipes, fullness usually comes quickly.

You want to rate your satiety after each meal, and you should aim to stop at a fullness level of 8 out of 10. Never eat until 'stuffed.' Ending up stuffed tells you that you are not aware of when enough is enough. Trust that your body knows the concept of 'enough,' and with real food this begins to come naturally.

How to build a meal

It's very simple. As you look at your breakfast, lunch, snack, and dinner, you need to see the components of a healthy diet: protein, healthy fats, vegetables or a bit of fruit. If you exercise intensely, and you don't have weight to lose, it's ok to also include some starchy, or direct, carbohydrates.

Thus, as you look at your plate, you may see a salad with olive oil dressing, a piece of fish, grilled vegetables, and half an avocado. Wash that down with a glass of sparkling water with some lemon and you have lunch.

For some great menu ideas, see our sample menus at EatMoveLive52.com/30Days.

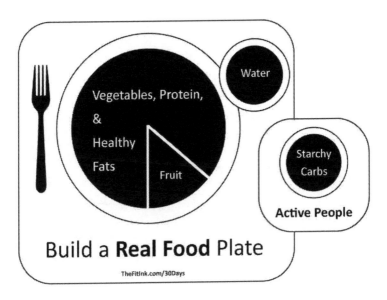

- **Vegetables, Protein, & Healthy Fats** – Focus on these as your primary sources of food, and don't worry about how much of each.

- **Vegetables** – Eat them raw, steamed, grilled, in soups, stews, purees, etc. Eat all colors and varieties.

- **Protein** – Choose meat, sausage, fish, eggs, cheese, etc., or a combination.

- **Healthy Fats** – Many protein sources already contain healthy fats, but you can also use butter or coconut oil for cooking, olive oil for dressings, nuts for salads or snacks, and avocado and bacon make great toppings.

- **Fruit** – For flavor or in small amounts, but not as a central dish. If you're trying to lose weight, watch your fruit intake.

- **Starchy/Direct Carbs** – Only in small amounts, and only if you're exercising hard or not concerned with losing body fat. After the first 30 days, this can change.

Consider these simple formulas

It's not that hard once you get used to eating this way, but try to remember these simple formulas. This is as hard as the math will get in this book...

Protein + Vegetables + Healthy Fats = Healthy Choices

Fruit + Starchy Carbs = Healthy, but optional, and often not optimal if you're 'on a diet.'

Myth: "No one ever got fat from eating fruit"

Not true, but it sure sounds like it should be!

We're often asked why we limit fruit, as it's a natural, healthy, 'real food.'

True, but remember that all calories and foods count, and the body doesn't discriminate much.

For many people, fruit isn't satisfying (it's the sugar), and leaves them just as hungry as before the fruit, leading them to eat again.

If they eat again, now they've overeaten, even if it all started with a 'healthy' snack of fruit.

Breakfast ideas

Breakfasts are not limited to breakfast foods	
Eggs + ½ avocado + sausage + tomato and cucumber	Eggs + cheddar cheese + mushroom and onion scramble topped with salsa
Greek yogurt with blueberries and handful of nuts	A frittata or crust-less quiche
Scrambled eggs and bacon plus baby carrots	Cottage cheese with pineapple, handful nuts
Steak and eggs, plus fajita vegetables	Omelet with peppers and guacamole
Leftover pot roast and grilled vegetables	Leftover ham, avocado, and vegetables
Cold chicken and leftover veggies	Whey protein pancakes: mix 2 eggs with 1 scoop of whey powder, and cook in coconut oil; serve with some fruit
Whey protein shake: scoop whey, cup water, slice pineapple, ½ avocado, and spinach	Sausages, peppers, and onions, topped with pasta sauce and a bit of cheese

Lunch ideas

Often packed yourself and made of dinner leftovers	
Large salad: spinach, tomato, bell pepper, shredded beef, grated cheese, olive oil and olives	Lettuce wrapped double burger with mustard, and apple on the side
A chicken breast, and tomato soup with parmesan	Meatballs with tomato sauce, grilled eggplant and zucchini
Pork roast with carrots and parsnips, Caesar salad (no croutons)	Meatloaf, coleslaw and handful of berries
Spaghetti squash with sauce Bolognese, cream of spinach soup	Stuffed peppers (ground beef and veggies inside) and broccoli and cashew salad
Meatballs and raw veggies	Fajita bowl (meat, peppers, onions, avocado)
Sausages (hot or cold), a chunk of cheese, and a small piece of fruit	Tacos in lettuce instead of tortillas
Vegetable soup and a side of roast chicken	A chicken bowl, with veggies instead of rice

Dinner ideas

Eat at home as often as possible and be careful with restaurant choices	
Tri tip with green beans and yams	Green salad, steak with cream of spinach and steamed carrots and broccoli
Bacon wrapped meatloaf, cream of cauliflower and parsnips	Meatball soup, taco salad with carnitas meat
Bunless California burger (beef, cheese, avocado) and green salad	Meatball soup and a chopped salad
Grilled salmon with grilled vegetables and pesto sauce	Chicken soup, chopped tomato and cucumber olive salad
Chicken or shrimp stir fry with lots of stir fried vegetables	Roasted chicken drumsticks and roasted root veggies
Steak fajitas with lettuce cups instead of tortillas	Taco salad (meat, salsa, avocado, cheese, lettuce, peppers, and onions)
Omelet of eggs, meat, veggies, and cheese	Slow cooker pork roast, with stewed carrots, onions, and summer squash

Remember to check EatMoveLive52.com/30Days for more ideas!

What about snacks?

If you get hungry between meals, have a small whey protein shake, a couple of hard boiled eggs, some beef jerky or a handful of nuts. If you are really hungry, just have ½ of what you would normally eat for lunch – protein, veggies, fats, and all!

What about dessert ideas?

Stick with a cup of fruit. If you really MUST have dessert, have a piece of dark chocolate and savor it slowly. To quiet your sweet cravings at night, make a cup of aromatic tea, such as Yogi Calm or apple cinnamon tea. Once you are able to go to bed without eating a sweet evening treat, you will realize it's possible and easy to do.

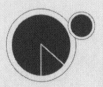

Hey, it's just a suggestion...

You can use our meal suggestions on these pages, or come up with entirely new ones on your own, just make sure you plan your meals so that they contain the main building blocks: protein, veggies, healthy fats, and the optional fruits or direct carbohydrates.

And what about drinks?

Hydration is of utmost importance. Shoot for half your bodyweight in ounces of water, so if you are 200 lbs., you are looking at 100 ounces of water. You can count tea in here as well. Make sure you are drinking at even intervals throughout the day, too, not just starting and ending the day with water. Some of our clients add a pinch of Himalayan salt to their water and swear by it for best absorption and energy levels, and it doesn't hurt to try.

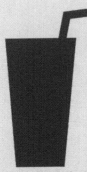

What about sweeteners and diet drinks?

Over the years, new artificial sweeteners, and even stevia, have made diet sodas and sugar free desserts more and more tasty. While it's true that these foods and drinks have less sugar and often zero calories, there are people who find that their appetites are actually stimulated by the sweet tastes, despite the lack of calories.

Remember, these 30 days are also about resetting our attitudes about food, and breaking food addictions and bad habits. Avoid them, and see how you feel in 30 days!

And what about restaurants?

Eating out on the 30 Days of *The Real Food Reset* is pretty easy. Almost every restaurant can cook a delicious piece of beef, chicken or fish on the grill and serve you a side salad or some steamed vegetables. Where it gets tricky is rich sauces and chilis laden with flour and extra sugar, so opt for no sauce, gravy or chili on your meats and burgers. We often order double bunless burgers over a bed of greens and a side of grilled veggies – pretty satisfying and all real food.

As far as fast food places go, you can still do the drive through you would just need to order bunless burgers and realize you may still be a bit hungry and may need to supplement with some nuts, fresh fruit, or veggies that you brought with you. If you are close to In-N-Out Burger or The Habit, their lettuce wrapped burgers are amazing, as are the Low Carb burgers at Carl's Junior.

Chipotle makes great veggie and meat bowls with healthy toppings and using naturally raised meats. El Pollo Loco serves chicken with sides of veggies.

It's possible to eat fast food and keep it as close to real as you can, so just do your best. If you feel stuck, send us a list of what's around you and we will help you come up with good and delicious lunches.

Never go empty for too long

Just like with your car, if you are running low on gas and keep driving past the good gas stations you may run out of gas right in front of a shady one, ending up getting poor quality fuel.

If you expect to find good food everywhere you go, you need to adjust your expectations, as sometimes you will have a choice between a gas station and a Starbucks, and real food is hard to get there (other than a larger-than-a-serving packet of nuts, and maybe a banana).

Go ahead and stock your car with jerky, nuts, apples, pouches of tuna and ready to drink protein powders (in a shaker bottle, of course). If you are stuck with no access to good food, at least you can have a small snack to hold you over. If not, you might overeat at your next meal, and we don't want that; overeating disrupts your hunger and satiety hormones and is a major barrier between you and your health goals.

What if I mess up?

None of us is perfect, and there will be mistakes, stumbles, and blunders, but we have a mantra or slogan that's worked wonders for us and our clients: "every meal stands alone."

Every meal, snack, food, or drink counts and empowers you to change the way you look and feel. Over time, you will change how you look at and feel about your food, but you simply can't let a mistake take you down. During the first 30 days, we do want you to be as strict as possible, meaning there are no planned cheat days or free meals, but coming up, we are going to cover the plan to allow you a little freedom. Hang tight!

In the meantime, don't worry if you make a mistake, and one meal isn't perfect; get right back in there and make sure your next meal is spot on. Put your choices in line with your goals.

Every meal stands alone.

If you fall off the bandwagon, get right back on it. If you fail at one meal, then allow yourself to fail at another and another, pretty soon you will be right back where you started.

Every meal stands alone.

"Every meal stands alone" is your reminder that one mistake won't take you down unless you let it. Don't let it. Every meal stands alone!

Ready. Set your mind. Go.

So far you have looked in your kitchen, done some shopping and some planning. You probably have a menu for 1, 3 or 7 days and you feel ready to start. This may have taken you a day or a week, but remember that it's important to prepare before a big game.

We covered how to prepare your fridge and pantry, and how to bulletproof your menu. It's time to look at how you prepare your mind.

Go back to your starting motto: "In 30 days I am leaner, I feel great, and I am more muscular than ever!" Whatever your motto is, write it with big letters, read it and believe it. It's cool if you can share it with your spouse or best friend and have them repeat it back to you. This technique of setting your mind on a goal is very powerful and was taught to us by our friend Bobby Fernandez, a CHEK holistic lifestyle coach. Hearing it in your friend's voice makes it very real and helps you solidify it in your mind.

Next, set a morning and evening ritual. Every morning for these next 30 days, open your eyes, smile and think of what your day is going to look like. Imagine your breakfast, your cups of water, how you order lunch at the cafeteria, how you go to your workout, the way you prepare dinner with your family. Oftentimes, your day is going by very fast and you may be overwhelmed with the tasks at hand, so having played the food scenario in your mind makes your plan easy and stress-free to follow.

At night before going to sleep, look back on your day and think about the great food choices you made, congratulate yourself on compromises, on amounts of food you ate, on remembering to drink water. If there is a place you slipped, like eating a donut that's not a part of your plan, think about ways you could have handled that situation differently. Think about positive changes you noticed from eating better and write them down in the chart in the next section.

All things NOT food

This month will rekindle your interest in real food and set you on a path of better health. Even though nutrition is an integral part of your journey, it plays a role in a much more complex and intricate system. Your health is influenced not only by what you eat, but also by how much you move, how you handle the stresses of life and how you recover from them, so we will go over a couple of 'extra' steps you may want to take over the next 30 days. By all means, do start with the food, and add these as you find appropriate for your life and goals.

Sleep

The average American is sleeping 20% less than in the 60's. That means that we are all losing a night's worth of sleep each week. It's not scary until you realize that sleep is how we recover from stress, manage hormones and enzymes, and make sure that our immune system functions optimally. There is a whole school of thought blaming lack of sleep for the epidemic of modern ailments, such as diabetes, heart disease, autoimmune disease and cancer, but suffice to say, if you are looking to improve your health through nutrition, making sure you have quality sleep is very important.

Start winding down for sleep at least an hour before your bedtime, dimming lights and turning off bright computer, TV and tablet screens. Sleep in a fully dark and well aired room. For those of you that find they wake up less than recovered, some magnesium glycinate may be a good supplement to take right before bed.

For most people 8 hours is a good sleep goal, but if you are only sleeping 5, maybe working on getting 6 is a good first target. I highly recommend getting a free profile over at Dan's plan (dansplan.com). Dan's Plan is a free platform that lets you log the times you go to bed and get up and calculates how close you are to your sleep goals. It also comes with free diet advice and recipes very close to what's in *The Real Food Reset*, so it's a great complement to our program.

Another way to track sleep is by using an electronic tool like the Fitbit (fitbit.com), which you wear on your wrist while you sleep. In the morning, it syncs with their online system and lets you know how long you slept, plus how many times you stirred.

Exercise

Movement is the missing element for so many of us. We are pinned to office chairs, computer screens and car seats, and then we go to the gym to make up for it.

The truth is that the body is a machine that functions optimally only when we move, and that means daily whole body movement. That includes walking, and lots of it when you can, hiking, working around your house and in your yard, playing with your kids, then doing some exercise on top of it.

"You can't out-diet a sedentary life" - Angelo Coppola, HumansAreNotBroken.com

For the next 30 days we want you to do something every day. Ideally, I would like you to walk at least thirty minutes, optimally sixty. On days when you are going to the gym, please still try to walk. Not a big fan of gyms? You can do some higher intensity training at home, using training programs like the ones in the New Rules of Lifting Supercharged, by Lou Schuler and Alywn Cosgrove or our time saving one dumbbell workout, The No Time To Workout Workout.

To sum up – walk thirty to sixty minutes a day, and on days when you weight train still try to do some walking. Not a fan of weights? Stretch or do yoga, but move your whole body 3-4 times a week on top of your daily walking (yes, DAILY!).

Supplements

We are not big supplement pushers. We believe you can do very well with just a multivitamin, an omega 3 supplement from fish oil, and some magnesium if you are having trouble recovering from your day. In winter, some of our clients take vitamin D. Other than that, we rely on real food to get most of our nutrition.

Please consult your doctor or nutritionist about your own supplement regimen and never take supplements randomly. During the 30 days of *The Real Food Reset* we recommend you take 2000-3000 mg of omega 3 (EPA+DHA

combined) from fish oil, as long as your doctors says it's
ok.

How to track your weight progress

Weight isn't everything. In fact, we often remind
people who 'want to lose weight' that they probably want
to lose *fat*. Still, sometimes you have to use the words that
people use, and weight is what's talked about.

Also, while fat loss is a primary goal, for most people
with fat loss goals, the weight *does* often need to come
down. It's rare that someone needs to lose fifty pounds of
fat and doesn't also need to lose weight, too. Swapping
fifty pounds of muscle for fifty pounds of fat is unlikely to
happen.

For most of our readers, fat loss and weight loss are
important, but we realize that some of you might be in this
for the health, and actually want to *gain* weight!

Either way, once you start to make changes to your
lifestyle and you start to feel better, lose weight, or gain
weight, you will want to be able to track your progress.

Let's start with your weight, which is simple to track.
...or is it?

Weight and fat tracking

You have several options to track your bodyweight,
your fat loss, and your lean body mass (the stuff that's not
fat). You might think it's as simple as stepping on the scale,

but as many dieters have found over the years, it's not always that simple. In the next few pages, we'll talk about the scale, why it's not always awesome, plus some other, often better alternatives.

The Scale

Pros – It's inexpensive and easy to use. It is also the one tool that you have used since childhood, so you probably already have a pretty good idea of what weight feels good to you.

Cons – The scale doesn't provide you with information about body composition, i.e. how much of your weight is fat and how much is muscle. If the scale isn't moving, and you don't know that you might have gained muscle, you might think your plan isn't working. Your scale doesn't know about water retention, a woman's period, dehydration, bowel movements (or lack of), etc.

How to use it – Your weight can vary on any given day, depending on the food and liquids you had, the amount of rest you got, whether you recently exercised or not, and more. To help with this issue, don't weigh every day. Instead take your weight only a few times a month, but when you do, weigh yourself on three consecutive mornings.

Weigh just after you have been to the bathroom and while wearing minimal and similar clothing. At the end of the 3 days, average your weight. This is your current weight. Do this every two weeks to know how you are progressing.

With this method, even if your actual weight isn't exact, you can at least track the trend, which you hope is going in the right direction.

Body fat scales

In general, we don't recommend these, as they are very unreliable; both in determining your actual body fat percentage *and* in seeing trends.

Pros – Body impedance scales *try* to calculate the percent of fat mass that you carry and provide a rough estimate of it without having to use special tools or pay someone to calculate the percentage of body fat for you. Used properly –and using the same averaging system as we outline for regular scales – you can often see trends in body fat percentage and weight.

Cons – Body fat scales give a range of inaccuracy that can vary between 3 and 10 percent. It's very hard to use them to accurately gauge progress or true body fat percentage. Make sure to use the same rules as with the regular scale; every two weeks, same time of day, same clothes, three day average, etc.

How to use it – Use your scales in the morning, on an empty stomach, ideally after eating and drinking the same foods and liquids the night before. Make sure you wipe your feet well before each testing. Ideally, you want to test yourself only a few times a month, but when you do, weigh yourself on three consecutive mornings, using the average of your three subsequent measurements.

Note that there are handheld devices that work similarly to these scales (body impedance), and they will have most of the same benefits and drawbacks.

Measuring tape (girth measurements)

Pros – It's inexpensive and easy to take your girth measurements at any given site. It is a reliable and consistent tool.

Cons – Girth gives little information of the quality of the tissues. You may have gained muscle and lost fat and you would measure the same circumference.

How to use it – Measure the following sites: calf, mid-thigh, hip, waist, chest and bicep (relaxed). Sum up all the measurements and write down the number. Take measurements every two weeks, preferably early in the morning. Note that your waist measurement will often be the quickest to decrease.

Body fat calipers

· **Pros** – They are the most widely used and one of the most accurate handheld ways of measuring body fat. After measuring skin folds on specific spots on the body, the numbers are entered into a formula. The result is the user's body fat percentage within a 3 percent margin of accuracy. Calipers also allow you to track local fat reduction in certain spots, so you know where your stubborn fat areas are.

Cons – It takes at least 100 measurements before you become good at pinching the sites in the same way. You may need special math skills, access to a computer, or complex charts to translate the skin fold measurements into your final results.

How to use it – Option one (recommended) is to find a good personal trainer who can do the measurements for you. Even then, try to use the same personal trainer every time, because even they vary by technique.

Option two is to do it yourself. You may need help for the sites on your back and triceps.

Whatever you choose, use a personal trainer or your own caliper kit that uses the seven site Jackson/Pollock method and formula for the highest accuracy. Take each site measurement three times before you enter each number into the formula, using the average of each site.

Take your subcutaneous fat measurement once a month, preferably before exercise and when your body hasn't been exposed to temperature extremes.

Before and after pictures

Pros – They are one of the most accurate ways to see muscle development, posture improvements, as well as fat loss. One client even noticed that his acne had improved because of progress pictures! Even if the scale isn't budging, pictures can tell a different story.

Cons – You need someone else to take the pictures or a timer on your camera. Having a friend take the pictures can be intimidating, but remember that the pictures will get better month after month. If you have a friend doing the 30 days with you, then take each other's pictures.

How to use it – Always take pictures in the same clothing each time, such as a bathing suit. Take them in similar light and surroundings. Take front, back, and side views.

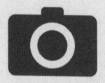

Regrets on being camera shy

Hi, Roland here... I still regret not starting with progress pictures, and I really struggled to notice progress at times. Pictures would have really helped with my motivation. Also, remember, those before and after pictures that you see on the internet all started with a before picture.

Choosing your method

Choose a method that is easy and accessible to YOU. We have found that a combination of the simple home scale, pictures, clothing fit, and the measuring tape to often be the best.

How to track your 'health' progress

The "30 Days of Real Food" and *The Real Food Reset* were inspired by our clients, and while some of them are looking to lose weight, a lot of them just want to shake sugar addiction, figure out if food is causing migraines, runny noses, brain fog, or anxiety. The trouble is, that unlike reading the scale and seeing that you lost ten pounds during week one, a lot of those symptoms are hard to track.

There's also an opportunity for progress in areas *other* than weight, fat, and muscle. Our readers have reported feeling better in general, but specifically better in things like acne, asthma, better sleep, joint pain, gas, digestion, and more.

Anecdotal evidence or not, they are seeing, and feeling, progress!

To make changes stand out more when they do occur, we have included a simple chart to help you evaluate your progress during the 30 days of *The Real Food Reset*. Day by day, rank yourself in the various categories using a scale of 1 to 10 (10 being most awesome), plus you can also record your bodyweight, if desired.

You can download a printable table of this chart from our website; EatMoveLive52.com/30Days

The Real Food Reset Symptom Tracker

You might notice that we say 30 days, but show you a 7 day chart. When you download the forms, you will be able to print off a full 30 day version, but it simply won't fit in this little book. We hope you get the idea, and we encourage you to download the full version of the chart and follow along.

Symptom/ Day	Monday	Tuesday	Wednesday	Thursday	Friday	Saturday	Sunday
Sleep quality	5	5					
Mood	7	8					
Exercise quality	7	8					
Brain function	5	5					
Work performance	4	4					
Thinking about food	9	7					
Digestion	3	4					

Mucus	5	5				
Runny nose	10	10				
Watery eyes	8	8				
Headaches	5	9				
Brain fog	9	9				
Skin quality	6	6				
Fatigue	3	5				
Gas	4	6				
Bowel movements	4	6				
Weight in lbs/kgs	167	n/a				

Again, this weekly chart is just used to illustrate how the chart works, but the full 30 day version is available on our site; EatMoveLive52.com/30Days

What if nothing is happening?

Well, that depends on what's not happening...

If you're not losing weight, consider that you might be losing fat, but not weight. Fat weighs less than muscle, so if you're putting on some muscle and losing some fat, then you're heading in the right direction.

Don't focus solely on the scale, but on the pictures and measurements, plus how your clothing fits.

In the previous pages, we listed quite a few methods for tracking your weight loss, which should really be *fat loss* for most people. Sure, we are a culture used to seeing a number on a scale, but if you look awesome and the number is higher than you're used to, just flaunt your athletic body and forget the number. Either way, remember that the number doesn't really matter, but looking and feeling great does.

Also, using "The Real Food Reset Symptom Tracker" on the previous page, see how things are changing in other areas. Like we wrote earlier, our readers have noticed significant changes in skin condition, hair, nails, digestion, mood, sleep, and more.

Remember, you didn't wake up one day and find yourself overweight and feeling tired and sick. It took time to get that way, and it takes time to get out of it.

Focus on the improvements that you DO see or feel, and give it time.

Day 31 and beyond

So, here's the part where we try to convince you to both continue eating like you have been for the last 30 days, but also convince you to relax just a bit, and give yourself enough freedom to enjoy life, and the occasional dessert, again.

At this point, you've seen and felt some positive changes. Great, but remember that the hallmark of the unsuccessful dieter is *stopping* the diet after they've seen good progress.

In our experience, people overestimate their own willpower, and underestimate the lifestyle that got them into the overweight and/or sick condition in the first place. It's not uncommon to lose weight, relax, and then gain it back and then some!

My friend Lou Schuler, fitness journalist, editor for Men's Health magazine, and coauthor of the New Rules of Lifting Series of books reminds us that 95% percent of those who go on a diet regain the weight again. Only five percent manage to keep the weight off for longer than five years. Why? What happens?

What happens if I stop dieting?

If you think you can go back to the way you were eating before the 30 days, you're most likely forgetting how things were. You were eating foods that weren't doing you any favors; foods that subconsciously encouraged you to eat more, spiked your blood sugar, and caused organs and glands to squirt and spurt hormones that negatively influence your health and appetite. All of this made you fat and/or sick back then, and it will again.

Going back to that isn't really an option, is it?

Yet, living a life entirely without some of your favorite foods isn't necessary, either.

Can I reintroduce certain foods?

I hope you haven't been counting the days, waiting for the 30 days of 'Real Food' to come and go, just so you can eat all of the foods you've missed! It doesn't really work that way; at least it shouldn't. Just a warning, but after 30 days of really good food and hardly any bad foods, your gut will be in for quite a shock if you throw caution to the wind and just eat your old standby foods again. It's not uncommon for people to end these 14, 21, and 30 day diets with a cheat day, only to spend that night in the bathroom!

Most likely, you started on the 30 days to lose weight, and we hope you have. Along the way, though, you might have felt and seen other changes take place. Among our clients and friends who have gone through the 30 days, many have reported positive changes in complexion, digestion, stress, blood pressure, mood, and more.

Some didn't realize that these things were better until the full 30 days had passed and they started eating 'old style' again. Suddenly, they felt gurgles in their guts that they had never felt before. Some had new pimples pop up, or started dragging their way through their day again. They started to see that food might affect things other than merely their weight.

When you do choose to experiment with some of your old foods – and you will – do it slowly, carefully, and one food at a time. If you were to go out and eat a commercial pizza, which has a large amount of carbs, oils made from soybeans, grains, or seeds, cheese, lots of sodium and probably some questionable preservatives and flavor enhancers, you might get sick, but which food made you sick? (And don't say 'the pizza.')

When you eat a complex food with many potential irritants or ingredients, you won't know which one irritated you. You need a method to the madness; why, what, when, and how.

Why?

Why do you want to reintroduce these foods? Most likely you miss them, which is understandable. Many foods *are* delicious...

Some foods are restaurant, family, or cultural staples, and avoiding them is a hassle.

Most likely, you've made significant weight loss progress, and feel like it's time to give yourself a little dietary freedom, while still keeping things moving in the right direction. You most likely never felt sick from these foods on your previous diet, and you only jumped on the

30 Day Real Food Reset to lose weight. You may or may not feel different, now, but by reintroducing some of these old foods, you might just find out.

If you don't suspect any food issues or intolerances, you can start adding a few favorites back into your diet. Just do it slowly. Don't have a cheat day or a binge, as your body is used to lots of good food, and a big dose of bad all at once can have dramatic effect.

Start with adding a favorite, suspect item to a meal (a bun to a burger, for instance) rather than starting with a fast food feast (burger with added cheese, chili, a bun, fries, and a soda or shake).

Many people aren't aware that they even have an issue with a food, mainly because our modern medical system doesn't always want to see the link between disease and nutrition. In the Precision Nutrition article titled "How To Do an Elimination Diet," Dr. Bryan Walsh writes about the potential links that food might have to some of the following symptoms or conditions:

- asthma and allergies

- autoimmune disorders

- skin conditions

- arthritis

- atherosclerosis and other cardiovascular diseases

- neurodegenerative diseases such as dementia

- mood disorders

- ADD/ADHD

- narcolepsy
- addiction
- migraines
- kidney problems

That's quite a list, and it's not always obvious that they are food related, hence the long lists of medicines, creams, and salves that are usually prescribed, rather than dietary changes.

Dr. Walsh's full article can be found at precisionnutrition.com/elimination-diet.

Remember to keep a log

...and track how you feel

You might be surprised to know that many people only discover that they had a food 'issue' during their second 30 days, as that's when the troublesome food has been reintroduced.

If this happens, you can always go back to eating more strictly for a while, and then try the slower reintroduction approach, outlined in the next few pages.

Of course, **if you do suspect you have food issues** (Do you have any of the symptoms or conditions listed above?), then it might be best to take the elimination/reintroduction approach outlined below from the get go.

What, when, and how

· After you've completed your first 30 days, and you're ready to try something you've really missed, we suggest that you start with a favorite ingredient and add it back in very small amounts, then see how you feel over the next few days. Resist adding in additional ingredients until you have a good handle on that first one.

Once again, test the ingredient or type of food on day one, then see how you feel on day two and three, without actually eating more of that food. On days four, five, six, and seven, you can try a bit more, all the while keeping track of how you feel. Do not introduce another type of food until you've given this first food a complete week.

This is the time to really ratchet up your journaling, so be sure to print off another "Real Food Reset Symptom Tracker" at EatMoveLive52.com/30days.

If at any point you feel a negative reaction to a food, stop eating it, and go back to eating more strictly until you're better. You can test again to be sure (assuming it's a food that you're really attached to), or move on to the next ingredient for the next week of testing.

Yes, this takes a while, but it's a good way to narrow things down.

Everyone who eats has their own list of favorite foods. Every diet coach who's heard client stories of food intolerance has their own list of foods that seem most likely to cause problems. My advice is to carefully decide on your food reintroduction choices, based on how much you love them and how likely they are to cause issues.

Here's OUR list of foods that seem to cause problem (allergies aside) with our clients; it's not scientific, but neither is your list of favorites!

- Wheat/gluten

- Whole grains/grains

- Faux grains (quinoa, buckwheat, etc.)

- Legumes

- Dairy

- Vegetable oils (which can be one or more of soybean oil, corn oil, cottonseed oil, safflower oil, etc.)

- Sugars or high levels of carbohydrate

- Eggs

- Nuts and seeds

- Artificial sweeteners

- Nightshade vegetables (eggplant, tomato, peppers, potatoes, etc.)

Our list is not exhaustive, and you'll notice that some items weren't even on our list of foods to avoid during the 30 Day Real Food Reset (like nuts, seeds, and nightshades).

If you suspect an issue with a food or foods, it might be worth dropping those for a while, just to see if 'that's your problem!'

Symptoms

Many of the symptoms can be obvious, like diarrhea or gas, but other symptoms are more subtle, like insomnia, feelings of fatigue, acne, rashes, breakouts, the return of joint pain, headaches, bloating, sudden weight gain, a food 'hangover' or brain fog, bowel changes, GI distress, sinus changes, watery eyes, asthma. Keep in mind that there can be positive changes, as well as negative, so keeping track of how you feel, and comparing it to the trends in the previous 30 days can be invaluable.

When to get professional help

Of course, if you suspect an allergy, intolerance, auto-immune condition, or have experienced something like irritable bowel syndrome, chronic heartburn, diabetes, lupus, memory loss, etc. then you'll need to be extra smart about it, and probably consult a medical professional. Let us know if this is you, and we can help guide you to the right person. Galya can be reached at eatloveandtrain@gmail.com and Roland is rdenzel@gmail.com. We will be happy to help you find the right practitioner to help you.

Come on, live a little!

I'm sure you heard that once or twice during your 30 days, but it should have been pretty easy to fend off that friend, knowing that you only had a few weeks to go, but what about now? It's day 31, 47, or even 184? What do I tell my friends now? Can't I live a little? Yes, you sure can.

It's safe to assume that there are some foods that you really miss and want back in your life. We understand that completely, and we aren't angels ourselves. We enjoy several foods that you won't find on the 'good guys' list for the 30 days of *The Real Food Reset,* but we have strategies in place to make sure these favorite foods aren't doing us any harm. We have found ways to limit our 'less than optimal' choices, all while enjoying a little more freedom than when we were strictly following the 30 days.

By now, you've at least read about why, when and how to reintroduce certain favorite ingredients, and chosen one path or another, but ingredients are just part of the story. With weight loss and body composition a typical goal for most people, there's often still a need to limit things like calories, carbs, and treats, just to keep your weight going in the right direction.

In case we haven't said it before, one major component of good health IS keeping your weight in check.

We often speak to our good friend, Alan Aragon, MS, who is a terrific nutrition researcher, plus a professional performance and diet coach to high-level athletes, not to mention people just like you and me. Alan finds that many health issues are also tied to how much people eat, not just to what, so outside of eliminating those foods you've found to be bad for you, getting and staying fit and trim is also important.

Constant overeating can wreak havoc on your body's systems, leading to chronic inflammation, insulin resistance, dramatic blood sugar highs and lows, and much more. Our body is a complicated machine, but when you challenge it for a long period of time it can only take so much. Eventually, your health shows the damage right along with your waistline. Likewise, improving your body composition has been shown to help repair the damage that was done while you *were* overweight.

"A hypo caloric state in and of itself has been seen to impart lipid improving effects and improve many health markers, regardless of changes in dietary composition." – Alan Aragon, MS, AlanAragon.com

Translated into English, this means that when you are overweight, and start taking in fewer calories to lose weight, your health markers should show improvement. When we say "health markers," we are talking about such things as cholesterol numbers, triglycerides, blood sugar, uric acid, etc.

You see? Changing to better foods is still important! The 'battle of the bulge' (and good health) has multiple fronts.

The 90% rule

So, with all that said, one way to 'live a little,' yet keep things under control, is to follow the 90% rule. Keep things clean or more strict 90% of the time, and cut yourself some slack the other 10%. Can this really work to keep you healthy? Sure. Can it really work if you want to continue to lose weight? Yep.

"100% nutritional discipline is never required for optimal progress. The difference in results, between 90% adherence to your nutrition program and 100% adherence is negligible." – John Berardi, PhD, PrecisionNutrition.com

At its most simple, the 90% rule means that 90% of your diet should be according to the rules of the 30 days, while the remaining 10% can include foods that are not necessarily perfect for your goals.

If you eat about 4 times per day, you can have about three 10% meals per week to play with. Here's the math: ((4 meals per day x 7 days per week) x .10) = 2.8, rounded off to 3 meals per week of your '10% meals.'

You could use these 3 feeding opportunities to have cheesecake one night for dessert, have a burger and fries for lunch one day, and have popcorn at the movies later that week.

Keep in mind that dietary restrictions for allergies and intolerances don't get a pass just because it's a 10% meal. If you need to be gluten free, a gluten free bun might be okay, but a regular bun is still terrible for you. If you're allergic to peanuts, then you obviously can't have peanut butter, despite it being a 10% meal.

Simple, right?

On the surface, the 90% rule sounds simple, but there are people who seriously overthink it and others who really work the loopholes. Both groups are prone to failure, just in different ways.

The 90% rule is a philosophy or idea more than a hard and fast rule; it will mean different things for different people, but if you stress about it and analyze it from the macronutrients down to the micro, you'll likely end up frustrated and annoyed with the whole program and eventually give up. If you're the type to look at the rule and see how you can maximize your 'fun' instead of keeping the spirit of the plan, you're likely to derail your diet even more quickly!

Good = 10% of your meals contains items that you consider less than ideal for your health and fat loss goals. Example: instead of sweet potatoes and roasted chicken you have reasonably sized hamburger and fries.

Not good = 10% of your meals contain desserts, beer, a burger and fries, and one of those blossoming fried onions with spicy ranch dip. This 10% meal can undo all the good your 90% has done, so beware and be smart about it.

Terrible = 10% of your meals contain ingredients that are causing you intestinal distress or acne, flaring your auto-immune condition, or causing you to use your inhaler more often.

Some foods need a 100% rule

A few pages back, we talked about some logical methods of reintroducing foods. We know that there are some foods that you might not be able to eat again. You might have 'known' these foods were an issue for a long time, discovered it during your 30 days, or be about to discover it during the process of reintroduction.

It can be very sad and upsetting to find that a food doesn't agree with you, but sometimes it's necessary.

Allergies – Allergies are an obvious example, and people who are allergic to peanuts, nuts, fish, shellfish, nightshades, etc. need to give them up, and often be ultra-vigilant in their food selection and preparation.

People with coeliac (aka celiac) disease have issues with gluten, and need to be extremely careful with their diet, as well, whether they feel sick after eating a gluten containing product or not. While coeliac disease is not an allergy, it should be treated as one, as it's a very severe reaction, with long standing and far reaching consequences.

Intolerances – People who have found that they are 'intolerant' to foods have to decide how strict they need to be about avoiding them. Lactose intolerance might cause gas or bloating, as an example, but some people are able to have dairy in small amounts or infrequently without much of a problem, while others really suffer from small doses.

Trigger foods – Trigger foods are another category, altogether. Do you think your 30 days cured a sugar habit?

Maybe 90% adherence to foods with sugar isn't enough. Maybe you need 95%, 99% or even 100% on those foods right now. This might not be forever – As your body and mind heals, you should come to appreciate 'real food' more and desire highly processed foods less and less. Give yourself time, and 'gently' test yourself at 60 or 90 days.

Addictions – Drugs and tobacco aren't the only things that you can become addicted to; food can be addicting, as well. While many people shake their heads like this isn't possible, consider the difference between a drug and alcohol, for instance. They aren't all that dissimilar, are they? Now, what's the difference between alcohol and coffee? All of these contain chemical elements that affect our bodies and brains to one degree or another, so why is it such a stretch to think you can be similarly addicted to even milder things, like tea, sugar, chocolate, or carbohydrates in general. Do we even need to go into addictions to things that aren't even ingested, like gambling or sex addictions?

What about manufactured foods, like mass produced chips? Can you 'just eat one?' Maybe, but if chips are your thing, it's hard to stop.

Addiction? Maybe on some level.

Yes, it's unlikely that a food addiction will have you so out of it that you'll wake up in a strange city, lost and alone, out of work, and sleeping on a naked, stained mattress (overhead, a bare light bulb swings). No, but it is likely that you'll get fat again.

Whether it's a food addiction, a newly discovered intolerance, or realizing that you can't restrain yourself with certain foods, it can be very hard to be faced with giving it up; whether it's forever or just for a while.

Losing a favorite food or ingredient can be painful, so focus on the positive changes that you've seen and felt instead. Know that you will come to enjoy other foods more and more, given time.

Maintenance (or, will this diet ever be done?)

What about 80%?

We find that even though 90% seems very restrictive at first, over time your cravings tend to change, and you don't look forward to the bad foods like you used to; at least not as many or not as much.

In addition, over time you will learn what foods are good for you and in what amounts. You might find that you can handle a serving or two of white rice per week without any issues, or that hummus, served as a side dish is not a problem for you. A big bowl of beans can bring you to your knees for days, but a couple of corn tortillas at Taco Tuesday don't seem to cause you any real harm.

These foods aren't optimal for you, but they might not be horrible for you, either. You may not feel like they should be fully counted in your 90/10%, so you can treat them differently or change your system to 80/20%, instead. Play around with it if you like, just keep monitoring your progress, and if you find that things are moving in the wrong direction, tighten things back up! Go back to a full 90/10% for a while, if not going *full* bore on another 30 days of *The Real Food Reset*, one more time, living and eating at 100/0% for a while, and reminding yourself just how good you felt when you were eating right.

Have a plan

As we wrote in our first book, 'Man on Top,' you always have to have a plan, whether it's a plan to lose weight, get stronger, get bigger muscles, or even to maintain your weight. ...and when you find your Plan A to be frustrating or not working, don't just abandon it, make a Plan B. While Plan B is in the works, stick with Plan A until you're ready to go.

If you have or develop an interest in fitness or nutrition, a good Plan B might be easy to find, as you'll enjoy reading fitness and nutrition books, subscribing to the blogs of your favorite trainers, and listening to nutritionists and dietitians on their podcasts, but not everyone will have those same interests.

Some people want help to find their Plan B, just like they did in reading Plan A; this book. We can certainly help with that, too. Visit the 30 Days Resources page at EatMoveLive52.com/30Days, and you'll find recommended reading, blogs of our favorite trainers to get you started, and even links to some great podcasts! If you want personal help, you'll also find links to our email addresses and Facebook pages there; contact us. Please!

Wouldn't you like to know exactly what to do to overcome your battle with food?

Don't you want to see yourself in the body you deserve?

If you've tried it alone and it's not working, a few sessions of coaching will greatly help your program!

Join the community

In our daily roles as health and nutrition coaches, we both lead small team challenges, in real life and online. Many of our team members are in America, but we have people playing and eating along with us all over the world!

One reason that we LOVE bringing people with a common goal together is that there is no power greater than the powers of community, family, and friendship when you are making a change or overcoming an obstacle.

As a community, we support each other, drag ourselves out of those diet holes, and celebrate each other's successes.

Stay connected

Studies show that a support system leads to a greater chance of long term success, so let's do this thing!

The very best way to stay connected with us is via email. You can call it a newsletter, but that makes it sound fancy, and it's really not. It's more like *us* sending an email to *you* every once in a while. We share stories, recipes, news, and updates with you, our readers.

Our email signup is at eatmovelive52.com/email

We also have a pretty active group on Facebook, and we'd love to see you there!

In the group, you can meet others with an interest in Real Food, find inspiration, recipes, tips, and be able to share your own real food adventures with others!

Facebook.com/RealFoodGroup

We'd love to have you in the group!

EatMoveLive52 & Real Food Resources

EatMoveLive52.com

Facebook.com/RealFoodGroup

EatMoveLive52.com/30Days

Contacting the Authors

If you want to connect us directly or privately, you can find Galina and Roland at:

Galina Denzel

eatloveandtrain@gmail.com

Instagram.com/GalinaDenzel

Roland Denzel

rdenzel@gmail.com

Twitter.com/RolandDenzel

Instagram.com/RolandDenzel

Other works by Roland & Galina

Eat Well, Move Well, Live Well – 52 Ways to Feel Better in a Week

Man on Top –Lose Fat, Get Fit, and Control Your Weight for Life

25 Minutes to Fit – The Quick & Easy Workout Plan for losing fat and getting fit in less time than you think!

Fit Mommy Secrets - The training manual that will give you everything you need to get back in shape after giving birth.

All available at EatMoveLive52.com/books

Book Updates

For updates on this book and our other projects, sign up for our email updates at EatMoveLive52.com/email, and get access to free resources and alerts on upcoming projects.

Acknowledgments

For help above and beyond the call of duty, a big thanks goes out to Pamela Lund, Debbie Hornburg, Anthony Sayers, Jesus, Doug Kartio, Ron Zissler, Andrea Feucht, Zacharie Quin, Ingrid Marcum, Alison Ross, Danny King, Rosie & Sean Henderson, and Wendy Welch!

Attributions

Reset Icon courtesy of EndlessIcons.com.

Many of the icons included in this book are courtesy of TheNounProject.com.

Carrot – svg_4475 as yourextralife.com, Chicken leg – noun_project_7789 as Marco Olgio, Dinosaur – Designed by Kyle Sasquie Klitch from The Noun Project, Bread – Designed by Jakub Ukrop, 2012, Bread – Bruno Gätjens González, from The Noun Project, Milk – Designed by Scott de Jonge from The Noun Project, Fruit – Designed by Jayme Davis from The Noun Project, Farmers Market – Designed by Cezar de Costa Area of organic fair 2013, Drink – Designed by Spencer Cohen from The Noun Project, Camera – Designed by Dave Tappy 2011, Genetics – Designed by Unknown Designer, Collaboration by Jack Biesek, Gladys Brenner, Margaret Faye, Healther Merrifield, Kate Keating, Wendy Olmstead, Todd Pierce, Jamie Cowgill & Jim Bolek United States 2004

Made in the USA
San Bernardino, CA
02 January 2020

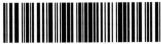